Mental Health and Later Life

The mental health needs of older people are all too often overlooked or put down to the inevitable consequences of ageing. This textbook will make it much easier for health, social care and third sector workers to identify, treat and support the needs of this population.

The book takes an interdisciplinary team approach and sets the scene by looking at different practice contexts in the United Kingdom and the increasingly important role played by social care in addressing the mental health needs of older people. A number of more clinically focussed chapters then cover:

- Mental health promotion.
- Anxiety and depression.
- Ageing and psychosis.
- Alcohol and dual diagnosis.
- Dementia.
- Later life liaison services.
- Complex and enduring mood disorders.

Each clinical chapter makes use of extended and detailed case studies which illuminate the Team's role in the assessment–intervention–evaluation cycle and ensure the text's application to practice. Service user and family perspectives are drawn on throughout and current practice exemplars outlined. The final chapter distils key messages from the book and sets a number of key challenges.

Mental Health and Later Life highlights the rewards and complexity of working with older people with mental health needs and their families. It is invaluable reading for all those learning about, or working with, this population.

John Keady is Professor of Older People's Mental Health Nursing at the University of Manchester and holds a joint appointment with the Greater Manchester West Mental Health NHS Foundation Trust, UK.

Sue Watts is Head of Psychology for Older People in Salford with the Greater Manchester West Mental Health NHS Foundation Trust, UK.

Mental Health and Later Life

Delivering an holistic model for practice

Edited by
John Keady and Sue Watts

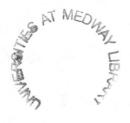

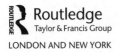 Routledge
Taylor & Francis Group

LONDON AND NEW YORK

First published 2011
by Routledge
2 Park Square, Milton Park, Abingdon, Oxon OX14 4RN

Simultaneously published in the USA and Canada
by Routledge
270 Madison Avenue, New York, NY 10016

Routledge is an imprint of the Taylor & Francis Group, an informa business

© 2011 John Keady and Sue Watts. Individual chapters, the contributors.

Typeset in Garamond by
Taylor & Francis Books
Printed and bound in Great Britain by
TJ International Ltd, Padstow, Cornwall

British Library Cataloguing in Publication Data
A catalogue record for this book is available from the British Library

Library of Congress Cataloging in Publication Data
Mental health and later life : delivering an holistic model for practice / edited by John Keady
and Sue Watts.
    p. cm.
Includes bibliographical references and index.
1. Older people–Mental health services. 2. Geriatric psychiatry. I. Keady, John, 1961– II.
Watts, Sue, 1957–
[DNLM: 1. Mental Health. 2. Aged. 3. Health Services for the Aged. 4. Mental Disorders–
therapy. 5. Mental Health Services. WT 145 M5475 2010]
    RC451.4.A5M433 2010
    618.97'689–dc22

                                    2010007756

ISBN 978-0-415-49428-1 (hbk)
ISBN 978-0-415-49429-8 (pbk)
ISBN 978-0-203-84475-5 (ebk)

Dedication

We have had the privilege of working with a generation whose lifetime of knowledge and experience was shaped in the turbulence, upheaval and opportunities of the 20th century. The strength and generosity of spirit they now bring to old age has been a constant source of inspiration. This book is dedicated to them, as well as to our respective families, managers, practitioners, researchers, educationalists and colleagues, who have shown us support and guidance throughout our time in this field.

John Keady and Sue Watts
February 2010

Contents

Illustrations

Figures

Tables

Contributors

Sube Banerjee is the Head of the Centre for Innovation and Evaluation in Mental Health within the Health Services and Population Research Department at the Institute of Psychiatry, King's College London. He is the UK Department of Health's Senior Professional Advisor on Older People's Mental Health and was co-lead on the development of the *National Dementia Strategy*.

Susan Mary Benbow is an Old Age Psychiatrist, family therapist and windsurfer who has worked in Central Manchester and Wolverhampton. She is Visiting Professor of Mental Health and Ageing at Staffordshire University. Her interests include the ongoing development of old age psychiatry services, and involvement of service users and their families.

Nora Bilsborough has extensive experience of working as a Community Psychiatric Nurse with older people, and has worked within memory teams since 1997; she joined the Salford memory service in 2006, taking up the post as Lead Nurse from September 2008.

Lorraine Burgess has worked with older people both in a general and mental health setting for 30 years. She is an Admiral Nurse in Manchester. Lorraine is currently working alongside her previous NHS Trust in piloting a dementia care pathway she has developed for the acute Trust as part of an action research dissertation.

Rachael Buxey is a Consultant Clinical Psychologist with older people as part of the South London and Maudsley NHS Foundation Trust. She leads the Psychological Therapies Service for older people in Southwark and also works as part of the older adults CMHT in North Southwark. She lectures for clinical psychology training courses in the London area.

Janet Carter is a Senior Lecturer in Old Age Psychiatry at University College London and an Honorary Consultant in Old Age Psychiatry at North East London NHS Foundation Trust.

Jenifer Chan is currently the Consultant Old Age Psychiatrist on Aubrey Lewis 1 ward at the Maudsley Hospital, Denmark Hill.

Georgina Charlesworth is an Honorary Consultant Clinical Psychologist with North East London NHS Foundation Trust, and a Lecturer in Clinical and Health Psychology of Old Age at University College London. She has worked in NHS mental health services for older people for 15 years.

Ann Crosland is Professor of Nursing at the University of Sunderland and Associate Director of the Centre for Translational Research in Public Health in the North East of England. She has extensive experience of mental health research in primary care settings and evaluation of community-based public health interventions.

Stephen Davies works as a Consultant Clinical Psychologist with older people at North Essex Partnership NHS Foundation Trust and as the Deputy Course Director on the Doctorate in Clinical Psychology at the University of Hertfordshire. He has an ongoing interest in the lifetime mental health effects of World War II.

Rachel Domone is a Consultant Clinical Neuropsychologist. She worked with Salford memory service from 2003 to 2009, during which time she completed her neuropsychology training. She continues to develop quality services for people with dementia in her new role with East Lancashire Memory Assessment Service, Lancashire Care NHS Foundation Trust.

Jane Gilliard established Dementia Voice, the dementia services development centre for the South West, and was its first Director. Jane was a member of the NICE/SCIE Dementia Guideline Development Group and the Working Group which developed the *National Dementia Strategy*. Jane is a Visiting Professor at the University of the West of England.

Julie Grainger is a Clinical Lead Occupational Therapist working within inpatient mental health services for older people in Wolverhampton. She is currently undertaking an MSc in Applied Ageing and Mental Health at Staffordshire University. She is passionate about providing the best possible service for older people with mental health needs.

Moganeswari Grizzell is an Advanced Nurse Practitioner/Research Sister and Visiting Lecturer at Wolverhampton University. She works in Wolverhampton memory clinic and is actively involved in the local Alzheimer's Society and her local church. Other interests include raising Alzheimer's awareness via roadshows, and services for people with learning disabilities/dementia.

Lee Harkness is a highly specialist Clinical Psychologist employed by Greater Manchester West Mental Health NHS Foundation Trust. He works both within a community mental health team for older people and a dementia-in-reach team. He works therapeutically with older people as well as providing support to families, carers and relevant professionals who care for those living with dementia.

Kadiatu (Kadia) Jalloh has been working in South London and Maudsley NHS Foundation Trust as a Psychiatric Nurse for eight years. As well as working with older people with mental health issues in the community, she has had experience of working in acute adult mental health and working with older people in nursing and residential care homes.

John Keady is Professor of Older People's Mental Health Nursing, a joint appointment between The University of Manchester and the Greater Manchester West Mental Health NHS Foundation Trust. John is founding and co-editor of the Sage journal, *Dementia: the international journal of social research and practice*.

Vanessa Lawrence is a Researcher within the Section of Mental Health and Ageing at the Institute of Psychiatry, King's College London where she has gained considerable experience in using qualitative methods in health services research.

Lorna Mackenzie works within the Newcastle Challenging Behaviour Team based in the Older Adult Psychology Service, Centre for the Health of the Elderly, Newcastle General Hospital. She has published a number of articles in the area of dementia care and challenging behaviour and has presented her work at national conferences in the UK and Ireland.

Jill Manthorpe is Professor of Social Work at King's College London and Director of the Social Care Workforce Research Unit. She was a member of the NICE/SCIE guidelines group, and is Associate Director of the NIHR School for Social Care Research. Her recent publications cover suicide in old age, support working, serious case reviews and social work training.

David Matthews is a Consultant Clinical Psychologist who has worked with older adults for 14 years, the last seven of which have been as the Clinical and Team Leader of the Croydon Memory Service. He completed his PhD at University of St Andrews and his current research interests include cognitive decline/dementia as well as service development and delivery.

Gillian Moss qualified in medicine in Manchester in 1980. She has been a Consultant in Old Age Psychiatry in Salford since 1988 and is consultant to the Salford Memory Clinic. She has extensive experience in working with people with all stages of dementia.

Joanna Murray is a Senior Lecturer in the Health Services and Population Research Department at the Institute of Psychiatry, King's College London where she teaches and applies qualitative research methods. She has conducted a wide range of studies of the experiences and needs of older people with dementia and their carers.

Faye Pemberton is a Social Worker, Approved Mental Health Practitioner and a musician, who has worked in Sandwell and Wolverhampton. She is currently a Team Manager in an Early Intervention Service. Her interests include using a variety of therapeutic interventions as tools for engagement, and challenging and redressing the stigmas attached to mental ill health.

Helen Pratt is an Advanced Practitioner in Dementia Care with Greater Manchester West Mental Health NHS Foundation Trust. Helen has worked with older people with mental health problems since qualifying as an RMN. She has worked within later life liaison services for Pennine Care NHS Foundation Trust for many years.

Rahul (Tony) Rao has been Consultant Old Age Psychiatrist at North Southwark Community Team for Older People, South London and Maudsley NHS Foundation Trust since 1998. He has clinical expertise in the assessment and management of older people with alcohol misuse and dual diagnosis and is a national champion for alcohol misuse in older people.

Lindsay River has been a lesbian activist since the 1970s. She has worked on health rights, carers' issues, and older people's rights. From 2003–09 she was Director of Polari, the older lesbian, gay, bisexual and transgender organisation, and undertook policy work, research and participation projects with older LGBT people.

Scottish Dementia Working Group is an independent campaigning group formed in 2002 by people with dementia who wanted to speak out for themselves. Membership is open to anyone with a diagnosis of dementia. The aims of the SDWG are to increase awareness, challenge stigma, improve services and influence policy.

Issy Scriven is a Trainee Clinical Psychologist at the Institute of Psychiatry, King's College London. She is currently conducting research into anxiety and sensitivity in young people with obsessive-compulsive disorder and autistic spectrum disorders. Her clinical interests include dementia care, child developmental disorders and mindfulness-based cognitive therapy.

Gyll Shields has worked in Older Adult Mental Health Services for ten years with a specialist interest in memory services. She has worked as a Clinical Specialist Occupational Therapist in memory services in Salford for the past three years, with clinical interest in early onset dementia.

Karin Terri Smith began working as a Psychiatric Enrolled Nurse in 1985, and much of her background is in working with people with dementia who have 'challenging behaviour'. She has been involved in some research studies and has had articles published. She has presented her work at challenging behaviour workshops.

Annie Wallace has 15 years' experience as a Health Improvement Specialist with lead areas in mental health promotion and problematic drug use. She is currently the Director for Public Health Curriculum Development for the North East Teaching Public Health network.

Richard Ward is a qualified Social Worker employed by the University of Manchester and Greater Manchester West Mental Health NHS Foundation Trust as a Researcher in Ageing and Mental Health. His research interests are in later life, especially dementia, discrimination, sexuality and embodiment, as well as inclusive approaches to participative research.

Sue Watts is Head of Psychology for Older People in Salford with Greater Manchester West Mental Health NHS Foundation Trust. She has been working with older people and their mental health issues since the early 1990s and now leads the memory assessment and older people's primary care mental health services.

Rosalind Willis is a Doctoral Research Student at the Institute of Gerontology, King's College London. Prior to this she worked as a researcher at the Institute of Psychiatry. Her research interests include the mental health of older people, informal care in old age, and ethnic diversity.

Foreword

Jane Gilliard

These are exciting but challenging times for those who are concerned about mental health in later life. In the future we may look back on 2009 as the year that made the difference; a watershed for care, service and policy configuration. The year started with the publication of the first *National Dementia Strategy* for England (Department of Health 2009a). This five-year plan sets out 17 objectives for developing services that meet the needs of people with dementia and their carers, whoever they are, wherever they are in the system and whatever form of dementia they have. There are many examples of care and support for people with dementia that are worthy of replication. However, for the most part, there is a huge mountain to climb to develop the care and support that works well for people with dementia and their carers, and for the systems that provide that care. People with dementia and their carers deserve care and support that is fit for purpose and fit for the 21st century.

The *National Dementia Strategy* for England (Department of Health 2009a) is not alone in its strategic vision. There is a momentum in the development of plans and frameworks to improve dementia care across the world. For example, at the 2009 annual meeting of Alzheimer's Disease International, a forum was held for those countries that are developing similar strategies, and representatives attended from Europe, Australia, Asia and North America. However, it is important not to be complacent; dementia strategies are the start of a process and not an end point. As an illustration, Professor Sube Banerjee recently published a review of the use of anti-psychotic medication for people with dementia which exposed poor practice and a need for additional work in the care home sector (Banerjee 2009). Contemporaneously, the Alzheimer's Society (2009) published a report on the care of people with dementia in general hospitals, which again called into question care practice and the confidence and competence of care staff working with this client group. Together, these two reports provide a wake-up call to commissioners and front-line staff, clinicians and providers of care. The 'old ways' of containing people with dementia and restraining them, whether with physical restraints or chemicals, are no longer acceptable. More enlightened attitudes, care systems and practice are necessary.

The end of 2009 also saw the publication of *New Horizons: a shared vision for mental health* (Department of Health 2009b). This cross-government programme of action aims to improve the mental well-being of people in England. It is age-inclusive and particularly addresses the needs of older people. With an emphasis on mental well-being and addressing stigma, *New Horizons* sets out an 'intention across a wide range of agencies to move towards a society where people understand that their mental well-being is as important as their physical health' (Department of Health 2009b: 7). The actions are grouped under a number of key themes: prevention of mental ill-health and promotion of mental well-being; early intervention; tackling stigma; strengthening transitions; personalised care; and innovation. The document highlights the importance of early intervention for older people. The Department of Health is working with several of the Royal Colleges, for example, to look at training initiatives to improve the identification of depression in primary care.

The *Let's Respect* campaign, developed by the Care Services Improvement Partnership (2006) [now the National Mental Health Development Unit], has proved a valuable resource in raising awareness of depression and delirium among staff working in general hospitals. It offers an example of how simple messages can make a big difference in practice.

The recognition of the mental health needs of older people in policy will require changes in practice. We are faced with many possibilities and opportunities and we should seize them eagerly in order to improve outcomes for those who use services and those who care for older people. Making change happen, though, requires a number of key elements. We need to review what we are currently doing and offer ourselves a critical challenge. We should keep and celebrate what's working well. We should familiarise ourselves with the new policies. We should look at what research tells us about what works and what delivers the outcomes that people want for themselves. We need to review the evidence base for the delivery of cost-effective services that offer good value. We need to scope what others are doing and learn from their experiences. At the same time, we need to allow opportunities for innovation. We need to be familiar with the demographics of our locality so that we can commission intelligently. We should be familiar with the local services that already exist, whether they are commissioned and provided by the local authority, health care organisations, housing providers, or the voluntary or private sectors. Then we will need to rise to the challenge of keeping what's working well; decommissioning what is no longer fit for purpose; re-commissioning services that meet the needs of those who use them; and, arguably the greatest challenge of all, giving people control of how they would like to be supported so that they commission their own care.

This book offers many helpful pointers to help work through such processes. Each author, an expert in his or her own field, reviews the latest policies (where appropriate) and outlines what relevant research has to tell us. They develop the evidence base. They give us case studies and practice examples.

There is often discussion and, at times, disagreement about how to ensure an equal balance between delivering services that meet the needs of people who have functional mental illness and those who have an organic condition. This compendium takes a broad view of mental health in later life. It encompasses the most common causes of both functional and organic mental illness. Importantly, it also addresses mental well-being and health promotion in mental health.

I commend the reading of this book to all those who have an interest in mental health in later life – those who are concerned about their own mental well-being, carers, students, strategists, commissioners, providers of care and front-line staff.

References

Alzheimer's Society (2009) *Counting the Cost: caring for people with dementia on hospital wards*, London: Alzheimer's Society.

Banerjee, S. (2009) *The use of anti-psychotic medication for people with dementia: time for action*, London: Department of Health.

Care Services Improvement Partnership (2006) *Let's Respect: the principles of best practice in the care of older people with mental health needs*. Available: www.mentalhealthequalities.org.uk/letsrespect (accessed 4 February 2010).

Department of Health (2009a) *Living well with dementia: a National Dementia Strategy*, London: Department of Health.

——(2009b) *New Horizons: a shared vision for mental health*, London: Department of Health.

Acknowledgements

We would like to thank Grace McInnes, Commissioning Editor, Health and Social Care, Routledge Books for commissioning the book and Khanam Virjee, Editorial Assistant, Health and Social Care/Law, Routledge Books for her invaluable help, guidance and patience during the book's compilation and submission. Our heartfelt appreciation is extended to each contributor, as without your expertise, time and commitment to both older people with mental health needs and to the project, there would be no book. Thank you. We would like to acknowledge our respective institutions, The University of Manchester and Greater Manchester West Mental Health NHS Foundation Trust, for their support and opportunity to work on the book over the last two years. Finally, but not least, a sincere 'thank you' to Eileen Woodhouse, secretary at the School of Nursing, Midwifery and Social Work, The University of Manchester, for her help throughout the compilation of the book and for her liaison with authors and the publisher. It could not have been done without you.

John Keady and Sue Watts

Glossary

A comprehensive glossary of relevant terminology, including lay descriptions of diagnostic categories, research nomenclature and key United Kingdom (UK) organisations can be found within the following document:

National Institute for Health and Clinical Excellence/Social Care Institute for Excellence (2006) *Dementia: supporting people with dementia and their carers in health and social care. NICE clinical practice guideline 42*, London: National Institute for Health and Clinical Excellence. Glossary pp. 374–86. Available: www.nice. org.uk/CG42 (accessed 12 February 2010).

The following is a brief glossary of key terms used within this book, which are specific to health and social care provision within the UK.

Care Programme Approach (CPA): This approach was introduced in 1991 and applies to the care and treatment of all patients in receipt of care from UK specialist mental health services. Professionals working for statutory mental health and community care organisations are required to work collaboratively to co-ordinate effective care for each individual. National standards for the delivery of CPA are in place. The terms Care Management and Case Management refer to related processes.

Care Services Improvement Partnership (CSIP): Launched in 2005 as part of the Care Services Directorate at the UK Department of Health, this organisation aimed to disseminate good practice and to help services implement national policy. It has now been superseded by the National Mental Health Development Unit (see below).

National Institute for Health and Clinical Excellence (NICE): This is an independent organisation which provides guidance within the UK on public health, health technologies and clinical practice. Their website provides further information. Available: www.nice.org.uk (accessed 12 February 2010).

National Mental Health Development Unit (NMHDU): This organisation was launched in 2009 and is responsible for a range of programmes funded by the Department of Health and National Health Service which aim to improve mental health and mental health services within the UK. It provides advice about research evidence and best practice, and supports the implementation of mental health policy. Their website provides further information. Available: nmhdu.org.uk (accessed 12 February 2010).

Social Care Institute for Excellence (SCIE): An independent registered charity, which aims to improve personalised social care services through the development, identification and promotion of knowledge about good practice in social care. Their website provides further information. Available: scie.org.uk (accessed 12 February 2010).

Single Point of Access (SPA): Also known as Single Point of Entry and Single Entry Point. This is a system which enables referrers to access a range of local health and social care services for individuals with mental health needs via a single service contact point from which initial assessment and signposting to related services will be arranged.

Introduction

John Keady and Sue Watts

At present, there is an intense policy, practice, education and research spotlight directed towards mental health and older people. As Professor Jane Gilliard states in the Foreword to this book, in the United Kingdom (UK) this is reflected in successive policy reports which have recently culminated in the publication of *New Horizons: A shared vision for mental health* (Department of Health 2009). This important document sets out a vision for a public mental health strategy [defined as 'the prevention of mental ill health and promotion of mental health': Department of Health 2009: 18] for the whole population whilst simultaneously addressing prevention, early intervention and treatment and a recovery approach from mental illness. Such strategies are to be placed within a life course approach (younger years–mid-adult years–older years), whilst also setting out a commitment for non-discriminatory services whereby older people are to have access to the same mental health services as are available to younger people, such as Crisis Resolution and Home Treatment services, assertive outreach services, Improving Access to Psychological Therapies and psychological services (Department of Health 2009: 84: Annex A). *New Horizons* defines older people as those over the age of 65 years (Department of Health 2009: 84), continuing a social and societal view on what it is to be 'old' that is embedded within our collective consciousness and aligned to social and public policy configurations of retirement.

Whilst a life course approach and commitment to service equality is to be welcomed, the *New Horizons* report (Department of Health 2009) contains some implicit assumptions about the design and delivery of mental health services that are still to be resolved. For example, is working with older people with mental illness the same as working with younger people with mental illness, the only difference being the passage of time?; do recovery-based models make sense when applied to older people?; how do people with dementia fit within a recovery approach?; is age attainment/division the best way to shape, deliver and fund a mental health service, or should this be constructed solely on the basis of need?; and what specialist evidence, training and skills exist in the preparation of practitioners to work in the field of later life mental health care?

These are searching questions and are not confined to the shores of the UK. Indeed, a European consensus paper on mental health and older people (Jané-Llopis and Gabilondon 2008: 6) found that older people (those over 65 years) have the highest suicide rates in Europe and that depression, chronic and painful illnesses and social isolation present in 71–95 percent of all completed suicides. The report also linked physical health and functional limitations to mental health problems in later life with socio-economic inequalities in health consistent amongst older people in the European Union. Interestingly, the report also found that the most pressing area to be addressed across member states was the reduction of stigma followed by, in descending order of priority, promoting active ageing and social participation; implementing prevention strategies: depression, anxiety, suicide, dementias, elder abuse; improving physical health; integrating services to support older people; undertaking carer interventions; improving the overall knowledge base; and capacity building and training (Jané-Llopis and Gabilondon 2008).

Contemporaneously, in the UK, this call for a more equal and inclusive agenda for older people's mental health was echoed in a high-profile and forthright consensus statement issued by the Mental Health and Older People Forum (2008), from which the following quote is taken: '**All** [original emphasis] of mental health in later life must be accorded the highest priority in terms of sustained vision, leadership and policy ownership, not falling through gaps between mental health and older people's policies. (p. 3)'

Mindful of this vision, as Editors of this book we have drawn on our practice, research and education experience of over 20 years each to respond to these priorities within a meaningful practice context: John during his role as a mental health nurse specialising in dementia care since the late 1980s, and Sue as a clinical psychologist working in older people's mental health from around the same time. Indeed, Sue remains embedded in practice in her role as Head of Psychology for Older People (Salford) at the Greater Manchester West Mental Health NHS Foundation Trust, whilst John holds a joint (older person's mental health nursing) appointment between the same Mental Health NHS Foundation Trust and The University of Manchester.

It is this complementary professional background and contemporary practice experience that has guided the philosophy behind the production of this book. As Editors, we are not trying to make grand claims and assumptions within the text about revolutionising mental health services for older people; rather, we have seen this book as an opportunity to hold a mirror to the mental health and later life field in the UK to see what works, why, and who is involved in multi-disciplinary care provision. Just as importantly, we seek to pose a question: where do we want to go?

Guiding philosophy of the book

As intimated above, this text aims to link a realistic evaluation of the complexities of living with a mental health need(s) in later life to the work of multi-disciplinary services and their response to such a need(s). Where it is appropriate, and in contrast to other texts available on this topic, we have encouraged contributors to write as a team in order to better reflect the day-to-day reality of providing later life mental heath care in primary, secondary and tertiary settings. Teams are asked to reflect on the focus of their expertise and service vision, and these were largely constructed around certain diagnostic classifications, such as later life psychosis, depression, dementia and alcohol dependency. Whilst each of these clinical chapters contains key information on demography, definition and key policy considerations of their respective diagnostic classification, the authors were asked to place the weight of their contribution on the sharing of a detailed case study(ies) so that authors/clinical teams had space to evidence their decision-making, outline the use and efficacy of assessment tools and describe applied interventions. A case study focus also allows the person(s) living with the diagnosis to be centre stage in the chapter composition and thus, in turn, to be seen as more than simply a label or a statistic. It is, in short, a textbook with a twist.

By compiling the book in this way, it is hoped that readers will be able to unpack some of the clinical decision-making attached to the case study(ies) and benchmark them against their own practice formulation/experience, as well as learn about the diagnostic classification. Moreover, it is also hoped that the case studies will be relevant to educationalists in helping prepare students for mental health practice whilst also providing a portal to allow more experienced clinicians time to reflect on professional practice. As Editors we would encourage and support creative use of the text and the messages it conveys.

We have also acknowledged the importance of social care and social interventions in the mental health care of older people; indeed, we have started the book with this very topic so as to maximise attention on user involvement and social care service development. Furthermore, when the contributors to this book were initially approached to take part, authors in the clinical context chapters (part two) were provided with a template to follow in order to provide heterogeneity within the overall shape and scope of the book. By and large this was followed by the majority of contributors but, as Editors, we have retained some flexibility within the provided structure and readers should be mindful of this as they make their way through the book. We did not want to hinder the creativity of authors in the messages that they wanted to convey in order to simply fit within a preordained structure. An example of this flexibility can be found in Chapter 8 (led by Rosalind Willis), where members of the Croydon Memory Service used their contribution to focus on generic working within their service and the implications that this has on general practitioner referrers and service users. This contribution includes qualitative research to evidence this flattened team approach and provides important messages for all multi-disciplinary teams involved in later life mental health services.

Before the overall contents of the book are introduced, we would like to say that we, as Editors, are responsible for the final structure of the text together with its omissions and limitations. On this latter point, for example, it could be argued that an additional emphasis on physical health care was necessary in order to allow a more complete discussion on the biopsychosocial model to emerge. Similarly, we drew exclusively on UK authors to inform the writing of the book and this was done in order to maximise the cohesion and messages contained within its pages. However, whilst these merits can be debated, we would like to think that the clinical and social situation(s) described in each of the case studies have some universally recognisable features. Whilst background policy, service and organisational structures for later life mental health services will differ from country to country, the key messages from the case formulations remain familiar. Like most textbooks, content was also restricted by a word limit and a need to stay true to the original aims of the book. Some hard decisions were therefore necessary in settling upon a final running order and we are mindful that not all readers will agree with our choices. However, we feel that the book provides the parameters for an holistic model for mental health and later life practice to emerge and in the common messages that are included in the final chapter of the text.

Structure of the book

The book is divided into three parts:

1 Setting the Scene
2 Clinical Contexts
3 A Way Forward

Part one of the book, Setting the Scene, comprises three chapters. The first of these chapters is written by Richard Ward with contributions from the Scottish Dementia Working Group and Lindsay River, ex-director of Polari. This opening chapter sets out the challenges and opportunities of user involvement and succinctly outlines the importance of applying and understanding a social model of mental health. This social care theme is taken up in the second chapter of the book, written by Jill Manthorpe. Using three case scenarios, as well as expert analysis on UK policy development and the social care role in older people's mental health, Jill provides a compelling account of social work practice and the holistic role necessary to fully address care interventions. The third and final chapter in part one is written by Ann Crosland and Annie Wallace, and focuses on mental health promotion in later life. This chapter provides findings on a number of mental health promotion and well-being initiatives conducted with the local population within the north-east of England. Despite a policy emphasis on preventative and well-being strategies in later life, there are relatively few examples available of such innovation. Transferable lessons from this work are shared within the chapter.

The second part of the book, Clinical Contexts, contains eight chapters and outlines multi-disciplinary working in older people's mental health care. The chapters in this section are mainly set out in a standardised manner (other than Chapter 8 as previously discussed) and follow a diagnostic classification pathway. The first chapter in part two (Chapter 4) is written by Georgina Charlesworth and Janet Carter, and addresses anxiety and depression in older people. Here, the authors outline two detailed case studies and psychological interventions, concluding that there is a need for new interventions to be developed that address key factors in late-life anxiety and depression. Next, in Chapter 5, Susan Benbow and her colleagues consider ageing and psychosis. Two case studies inform this chapter which involve teamworking and the challenges presented by negotiating a therapeutic relationship with users who lack insight into their psychosis. As these authors discuss, communication, co-ordination of treatment and the flexibility to tailor treatment plans to individuals and their families are identified as major issues in practice within this specific client group. The third chapter in this section (Chapter 6) is written by Rahul (Tony) Rao and his colleagues and considers the much under-reported area of alcohol and dual diagnosis (alcohol misuse and serious mental illness existing side by side) in older people. A detailed case study is presented that combines formal therapy, such as supportive psychotherapy, cognitive behavioural therapy and motivational interviewing, with practical help such as engaging with local resources. The next three chapters in this part of the book focus on people with dementia, although they use a different lens to view the experience. The first of these three chapters (Chapter 7) is written by one of the Editors, Sue Watts, and includes the contribution of her colleagues from the Salford Memory Assessment Team. Here, the role of memory clinics and their pivotal role in the early identification of dementia are considered, and a number of case studies are shared which provide an illustration of the complexity of this work. Chapter 8, by Rosalind Willis and her colleagues from the Croydon Memory Service, details the use of generic working within this influential and well-known service. Through a qualitative evaluation shared within this chapter, such a flattened team structure is demonstrated to be effective for referrers to the service. Completing the series of three chapters focusing on dementia care, Chapter 9 is by Karin Terri Smith and Lorna Mackenzie who describe the work of the award-winning Newcastle Challenging Behaviour Service and the focus on being alongside people with dementia who present with challenging behaviours in a care home setting. A detailed case study is presented in the chapter together with the team's approach to case for-mulation and intervention. The penultimate chapter in the Clinical Contexts section (Chapter 10) is written by Helen Pratt and Lorraine Burgess and is centred on later life liaison services and the delivery of mental health care within general hospitals. A composite case study, based on examples of care taken from a number of anonymised patient cases, is variously shaped and adapted to reflect the diversity of situations faced by such clinicians. Successful collaborative working emerged as a key aspect of the liaison role. The final chapter in part two (Chapter 11) is written by Stephen Davies and draws on an extensive case study to outline the problems of chronic low mood in late life and living with lifelong mood problems. A discussion around the importance and meaning of attachment theory is also presented.

The third and final part of the book is called 'A Way Forward' and is written by the Editors. This brief concluding chapter (Chapter 12) draws out four key messages from the whole book and looks forward to a new agenda for later life mental health care.

The start of the 21st century has seen the consolidation of a mixed economy of ser-vice provision in older people's mental health care where new cultures and ways of working, funding and commissioning are prominent. Indeed, the traditional belief that one service or professional has a lead and ownership of older people's mental health care has been eroded and replaced by a new language, a discourse of prevention, con-sumerism, involvement, personalisation and self-care. New watchwords for the dawn of a new century. However, whilst such a change of focus is to be embraced, what cannot be forgotten is that some older people experience mental illness that is complex, enduring and debilitating, and/or have simply aged with long-standing mental health needs. Skilled, co-ordinated and planned evidence-based care delivered through a trained workforce remains necessary. The spotlight should not shift too far from this ground.

We hope that you enjoy this book.

References

Department of Health (2009) *New Horizons: A shared vision for mental health*, London: Department of Health.

Jané-Llopis, E. and Gabilondon, A. (eds) (2008) *Mental Health in Older People*, Consensus paper. Lux-embourg: European Communities. Available: www.ec-mental-health-process.net (accessed 4 February 2010).

Mental Health and Older People Forum (2008) *A collective responsibility to act now on ageing and mental health. A consensus statement issued by key organisations integral to the support, care and treatment of mental health in later life*, London: Mental Health and Older People Forum. Available: www.mentalhealthequalities.org.uk/silo/files/consensus-statement-august.pdf (accessed 4 February 2010).

Part 1

Setting the scene

1 Between participation and practice

Inclusive user involvement and the role of practitioners

Richard Ward with contributions from the Scottish Dementia Working Group and Lindsay River, Ex-Director of Polari

Key messages

- Inclusive measures are vital to user involvement in order to avoid replicating existing inequalities in access to health and service care.
- Practitioners have an important role to play in strengthening user participation and can work together with users to tackle exclusion and discrimination against particular groups and communities.
- Adopting a social model of mental health within the involvement process can assist in tackling the structural barriers to the participation of service users.
- Taking account of the biographies of service users supports a better understanding of the cumulative impact of exclusion and discrimination upon their involvement in user networks.
- Making relations of power explicit within user involvement initiatives can support the development of empowering practice and help in the recognition of differences between service users.

Introduction

The participation of service users in the structures and processes of the welfare state is now widespread, although still far from systemic. User involvement has evolved politically from something tolerated at the margins of health and social care to an undertaking now required of both health and local authorities (Department of Health 2006, 2007, Dialog 2007). This shift reflects broader social and political changes as forms of democracy and citizenship become more localised and diffuse and the grand narratives of twentieth-century politics fade from view. As with much recent rights-based policy, participation has been introduced as an administrative duty on providers and straddles different cultures and disciplines within health and social care. It has the potential both to unify the provision of services and erode long-standing divisions between differing professional groups and the individuals they support. Yet, participation of service users is one of the least well evidenced reforms to recent policy (Campbell 2001), especially in terms of its outcomes (Carr 2004), and little detail is known about who gets involved or how (Bochel *et al.* 2008).

This chapter addresses three key questions:

1. What role can practitioners play in strengthening participation?
2. Why is inclusivity important to user involvement?
3. How can inclusive forms of participation best be achieved?

The discussion focuses on the challenge of developing inclusive forms of user involvement. Without inclusive measures there are few guarantees that participatory mechanisms will necessarily avoid the exclusions and inequalities that currently prevail in health and social care. Practitioners have a vital role to play in this process through enabling individual users and by ensuring the involvement process reflects diversity and supports difference. A case is made for looking beyond the way services define users according to presenting needs, to consider instead the significance of a broader social and biographical context as a basis for involvement. The idea of a uniform category of service user is questioned through reference to two case studies of user involvement with groups that have historically been excluded from the planning and provision of mental health services.

Practice supporting participation

Within the existing literature there are (at least) three ways in which user involvement has been portrayed:

- As a conceptual clash (Carr 2007) between a top-down set of policies and a so-called bottom-up social movement.
- As a spectrum of involvement activities where there is an emphasis on the heterogeneity of approaches and methods (Nolan *et al.* 2007a, 2007b).
- As one element on a spectrum of actions in which users are engaged (Campbell 2001).

Beyond these characterisations are a host of more sceptical standpoints, with emphasis placed on participation as a hegemonic system or technology by which policy-makers and service providers seek to legitimate their own interests (Harrison and Mort 1998, Carey 2009). Despite such an array of perspectives there has been a tendency to neglect the role of the practitioner, with limited thought given to where health and social care practice fits into the involvement agenda. Indeed, little evidence currently exists of the opportunities for practitioners to reflect on what user involvement means to them – either collectively or as individuals. Only recently have calls been made for the training and education received by practitioners to include skills associated with supporting user participation (e.g. Barker and Rolfe 2004, Postle and Beresford 2007).

Instead, two increasingly well-documented forces have been argued to drive user participation in the welfare system. One such force consists of often well networked, vocal and co-ordinated user movements. In mental health, this movement has worked to challenge entrenched beliefs, for example drawing attention to the socially located and constructed dimension to mental health difficulties while placing emphasis upon social attitudes to mental illness, stigma and other adverse conditions. Such emphases imply the need for a broader social agenda for mental health rather than individualised medical responses. By contrast, a consumerist doctrine in policy has promoted involvement as a route to improving services but has presented few challenges to existing structures or relations. In the context of this tension between top down policy and grass roots campaigning, where does the practitioner figure?

New working cultures

The only part of an organisation that many service users come into contact with is their individual worker or service team. Much rides on the quality of this encounter, and the extent to which the parties are able to develop a relationship in which professional expertise is put at the disposal of the service user's agenda.

(Braye 2000: 24)

The integration of health and social care creates new contexts and cultures for practice. Different professions are finding their working practices open to scrutiny as they seek to articulate and share their skills whilst establishing routes to collaborative working. In this context, Barker and Rolfe (2004) have called for the reframing of the nurse's role through a rights-based approach. They argue that mental health nurses are increasingly working in 'multi-disciplinary and community-based settings where they are both more exposed to social approaches and more able to take forward social approaches in their own work' (p. 366). Similarly, Carr (2004) has recommended that 'frontline practitioners could be usefully engaged in user participation strategies and benefit from a user-led training focusing on the practice and principles of user participation' (p. 273).

The move toward integrated health and social care provision has brought professional differences to the surface that have implications for user involvement. The rather more clearly set out and hierarchised knowledge-base in health has been perceived as disadvantaging social care workers (Gould 2006), whose working knowledge is often more tacit, context-specific and consequently more difficult to articulate or aggregate (Pawson *et al.* 2003). Yet the skills associated with social care approaches have been argued to lie at the heart of a move toward strengthening user involvement and the enabling of service users (e.g. Postle, Wright and Beresford 2005). This shift involves the recasting of the practitioner from the role of expert, defining user needs and deciding on their behalf how best to respond to that of a facilitator, working in partnership with users.

In respect to working with older service users, Thompson and Thompson (2001) describe this as a shift from a care of the elderly model to one of empowering practice. Integral to this is the need to challenge the effects of ageism and how they shape relations between practitioners and users, and the development of more collaborative forms of working that aid user decision-making and greater levels of involvement in the welfare system. The authors highlight three key features of practice necessary to this partnership style of working:

1 Interpersonal and problem-solving skills that raise confidence and self-esteem and challenge the effects of ageism.
2 An understanding of services, resources and other opportunities available to users.
3 The capacity to analyse complex social and personal circumstances and help identify ways of moving forward.

(Thompson and Thompson 2001: 66)

Why is inclusivity important to user involvement?

A compelling argument for user participation is that service users possess insights into their own needs, and a situated understanding of the services they access to meet those needs, which is otherwise inaccessible to providers (Beresford and Croft 2001). Within mental health provision, evidence of the incorporation of situated knowledge is beginning to emerge, signalled by a growing concern to ascertain user-defined criteria and outcomes as a means to develop more tailored forms of care and support (e.g. Perry and

Gilbody 2009). The challenge for such participatory approaches lies in how well they are able to take account of difference and avoid creating normative categories of service users.

All users are not equally well placed to participate, and face barriers to involvement that are comparable to those when accessing services. Yet there is limited commentary on how individuals are recruited or engaged by participation mechanisms. A review by Tait and Lester (2005) found that most mental health user groups are small, poorly funded and non-representative of minority groups or communities; while Webb (2008) has observed that where service user groups are active they are usually self-selecting and their forms of accounting to a wider public are often uncertain. In short, little is known about the patterns of exclusion that currently define and mark out the participation process within health and social care. Forbes and Sashidharan (1997) succinctly summarise this dilemma in the following way: 'A uniform notion of users implied by the current model, such as mental health users, older users or users with a disability is made possible only by ignoring the heterogeneity of users' (p. 492).

Forbes and Sashidharan (1997) also highlight a series of reasons for looking beyond the category of service user – summarised below:

- Users do not have a uniform relationship to services.
- Needs differ, as do experiences of a service.
- Broader social divisions shape access to and experiences of a service.
- Notions of need and risk are also shaped by a wider social context.
- Inequalities and divisions can be reinforced by services (for example, the higher levels of custodial and coercive forms of intervention employed with Afro-Caribbean mental health service users).

Such considerations highlight why there is a need for inclusivity in user involvement mechanisms, and underline the role played by health and social care in constructing the identities of service users while also upholding differences between them, both within and beyond service provision. An example that has particular relevance to mental health services for older people is the relationship between medicine and homosexuality.

The significance of a biographical context: older lesbian, gay and bisexual (LGB) mental health services users

Work conducted with older LGB people underlines the significance of taking into account a biographical context when such individuals access mental health services as well as in the development of participation mechanisms with older service users. At earlier points in their lives older gay, lesbian and bisexual service users were viewed and treated by psychiatrists and other medical practitioners as mentally disordered, a view supported by a longstanding concern within medicine to identify the cause of homosexuality. Only relatively recently was homosexuality removed from psychiatric diagnostic manuals. For older LGB service users such experiences form part of a wider context of discrimination, persecution and social exclusion that feature across many domains of everyday living, examples of which include:

- Family and education: possible rejection and estrangement from birth family and bullying in the school system.

- Workplace: harassment, exclusion and institutionalised discrimination affecting career prospects.
- Public spaces: violence, threats and abuse.
- Goods and services: formal and informal exclusion and discrimination, e.g. access to financial services.
- Relationship to the State and large social institutions (such as medicine, the church and the legal system): including condemnation by the church, the criminalisation of homosexuality prior to the *Sexual Offences Act* (Office of Public Sector Information 1967), and potential loss of custody of children.

This array of experiences underlines the importance for practitioners of taking into consideration a biographical context and, in particular, awareness of the cumulative nature of their impact upon the lives of older LGB service users. This context provides a basis for understanding a) the significance of broader divisions between service users, b) differences in their experiences of mental health services, and c) the role played by medicine in the labelling and stigmatising of LGB identities. Such considerations have direct implications for LGB user involvement in older people's mental health services and user networks.

A user-led investigation of older lesbian, gay and bisexual (LGB) people's experiences of mental health services: contribution from Lindsay River, Ex-Director of Polari

Polari was a voluntary organisation that ran from 1993–2009, with the aim of raising awareness of diverse sexualities and promoting good practice within services to older people. Between 2002–06 older LGB people were recruited to a participatory project and consulted on their experiences, which were shared (anonymously) with service providers and commissioners in three London boroughs. The project (see Davies and River 2006 for further details) found that mental health issues were a priority for many participants and that their needs were poorly met by services. Further research on older LGB people's experience of mental health services was called for and a scoping study was set up to examine the issues that arose for users.

The subsequent study (detailed in Wintrip 2009) uncovered a long history of negative experiences of mental health services on the part of those who participated. This included past experiences such as aversion therapy and the treatment of homosexuality as a mental illness – an experience considered by some to have damaged their lives in a far-reaching way – up to very recent and on-going instances of discrimination and violence. Users spoke of the lack of safety they had experienced and the prejudices they faced both from workers and other users in mental health services, and highlighted a need for separate LGB mental health user groups. The difficulty, for reasons of community safety, of involving LGB people in mainstream mental health service user/survivor groups were also outlined, and the users consulted seldom felt confident that existing user networks understood or were sympathetic to their specific needs.

The study recommended that mental health services take a clear and zero tolerance approach to homophobia from staff and develop strategies to address this amongst users to create safety for LGB users, particularly in acute mental health care. The lack of recognition and support for carers of LGB people with mental health issues was stressed, as was the need for all members of multidisciplinary teams to have comprehensive training on sexual orientation. Similar needs around training exist on issues of gender identity.

Though Polari has occasionally encountered successful one-off consultations with LGB people, run by statutory services such as a council or a health service, it is less common to find a statutory-run ongoing and sustainable user involvement group of this kind. However, sustainability was a major issue for Polari throughout its life. With short-term funding, staff were required to develop exit strategies and devote time to producing final reports, undermining efforts to search for new funding or pursue new recruits. Sustainable user involvement of minority groups needs ongoing funding and support to the organisations that work with them or are led by them.

With older LGB groups recruitment takes considerable time and effort. The project faced particular challenges in recruiting black, Asian and minority ethnic LGB elders and it was clear that extra time and resources were needed. Due to lower numbers, cultural and demographic differences, workers who know of the needs of these groups may need to become advocates for those who do not want to 'out' themselves. In our experience it is likely to be more effective to combine user involvement with social networking opportunities that may attract participants by meeting a real local need for sociability or by supporting older LGB people to form user-led campaigning groups.

Participatory and involvement work with older LGB people presents particular challenges with mental health service users and survivors, due to issues of trust and worries about safety that are likely to interfere with involvement work until the issues outlined above have been better addressed. Staff at all levels and user groups could work together positively to eliminate heterosexism, homophobia and transphobia wherever they might appear in the services, and co-create strategies to make wards, units and community-based resources safer for LGB service users. By creating a sense of greater safety, it is likely that new participatory and involvement projects will have a much greater chance of thriving.

Further reading on sexuality, ageing and mental health: McFarlane (1998); Smith, Bartlett and King (2004); Wintrip (2009).

Approaches to inclusive participation: consensus or conflict?

Understanding how modes of involvement may position service users, imply assumptions about them or shape their input is a key consideration for practitioners. The road to a more systemic presence for user involvement throughout the welfare system rests upon both tackling the barriers that currently prevent participation by certain groups and individuals whilst raising awareness of the mechanisms that best support inclusivity.

Nolan *et al.* (2007a, 2007b) outline the benefits of developing a diverse range of methods for engagement. The authors argue that a mix of approaches may better support involvement by groups and individuals that, to date, have been less engaged by existing mechanisms. As Frankham (2009) observes, this includes groups that are among the highest users of welfare services, such as people with dementia. Nolan *et al.* (2007a, 2007b) emphasise the potential for co-learning that comes from the relationship between researchers/practitioners and users. Such a relationship-centred perspective on participation underlines that responsibility for its development is shared between practitioners, users and at the service/organisational level. The authors conclude that it is 'productive to talk about creating a new shared world with a common set of concepts and values' (Nolan *et al.* 2007b: 196). It may be helpful to think of this as a consensus model of user involvement in which all parties or stakeholders are perceived as working for a common cause and with a shared interest.

By contrast, many within the existing user movements draw upon a conflict model as the basis for understanding the context of user involvement. For instance, Campbell (2001) argues that the language of partnership and common concerns conceal realities of different agendas, interests and imbalances of power. This view of the welfare system has led some commentators to assert that large-scale user-led and user-defined forms of participation represent the ideal goal. Larger networks of users may better reflect the diversity of users through a democratic structure. As an example, Beresford and Campbell (1994) draw attention to the emergence of a user culture within the disability movement that includes the production of different forms of art and the moulding of identities that stand outside of medicalised categories and labelling. This democratic, user culture model of participation holds particular potential for recasting relations within the welfare system. For instance, within the mental health movement, some users have redefined themselves as survivors in order to better communicate their experiences and distance themselves from the part of consumers of a service. Table 1.1 summarises the benefits of heterogeneity and of a user culture model as presented in the literature.

Applying a social model of mental health to user involvement

While user-led initiatives have disputed existing hierarchies in mental health provision, policy-driven involvement activities tend to incorporate service users into existing mechanisms in an add-in and stir approach. Simply appending user involvement to established systems has required users to participate in contexts for which they can be ill-prepared, unfamiliar with existing protocols and where they feel pressured to speak out on issues of which they have little experience or knowledge (Carr 2004). Such conditions can penalise individual restrictions or impairment and to date have led to certain groups, such as people with dementia, being largely excluded from involvement strategies. McDaid (2009) argues that mental health conditions cannot be ignored within participation mechanisms,

Table 1.1 The benefits of a heterogeneous model compared with a user culture model of participation

Benefits of heterogeneity	Benefits of a user culture model
Tailored to different levels of capacity/motivation for participation	Democratic (provides user representatives with a mandate)
Enables contributions from highest level users	Larger networks are better able to reflect the diversity of users
Recognises and supports differences between users	Greater political strength and influence in numbers
Addresses complex needs	More autonomous (so less open to influence by providers)
Recognises that user involvement can be adapted to serve different purposes and function at different levels of influence	Fosters an alternative discourse and construction of identities beyond medicalised labels and categories
Enables individual voices to be heard	Challenges broader cultural definitions, negative stereotypes and the stigma attached to being a service user

but, rather than leading to a focus on individual deficits, should prompt awareness of the structural barriers within decision-making forums. From this perspective, difficulties with concentration, stamina and other fluctuating capacities serve to challenge the normative expectations attached to events such as committee meetings, interviewing panels and other organisational routines. However, the question remains: what are the implications of such an approach in the context of services to older people?

Mechanisms for participation in mental health services for older people are under-developed compared with those of working age users, and older service users with the highest levels of need have been argued to be in a position from which little or no power can be exercised (Gilliard and Higgs 1998). The image of a vocal, well-networked mental health service user with a critical understanding of service provision and policy contrasts starkly with portrayals of older people accessing the welfare system, with low expectations of services and the likelihood to report high levels of satisfaction. As a group, older people are the highest users of health and social care services and yet their voices are rarely heard and little evidence exists of the impact of their involvement on the quality of care or the structuring of services (Cook and Klein 2005, Postle, Wright and Beresford 2005). A significant challenge to an evolving user involvement agenda is how high-level users of welfare services can be supported to have a voice in this process.

User involvement and people with dementia

At present, people with dementia are among those on the periphery of current mental health user networks and have tended to be excluded, often formally, from initiatives to involve older service users (e.g. Barnes and Bennett 1998). Only recently has a debate on how to balance safeguarding with empowerment begun to influence dementia care practice. Historically, people with dementia have been excluded from the planning and provision of services both collectively and as individuals, due to assumptions over their incapacity to communicate. Such routine exclusion has been described as cognitive disablism; a particular form of discrimination faced by this group (Ward *et al.* 2008).

Gilliard and Higgs (1998) warn that efforts to involve people with dementia can lead to artificial outcomes where 'no apparent mental or physical barrier is to be acknowledged in the pursuit of the authentic voice of the user' (p. 241). Increasingly, however, emphasis is shifting toward a social model of dementia which 'allows us to confront the ways in which we discriminate against people with dementia and marginalise them' (Care Services Improvement Partnership 2007: 12; see also Gilliard *et al.* 2005; Bartlett and O'Connor 2007). Such an approach signals the importance of involving users in ways that recognise but do not penalise impairment (Cheston, Bender and Byatt 2000). For practitioners this means working collaboratively to develop modes of involvement that accommodate fluctuating capacities and restrictions due to impairment while questioning the artificial barriers that prevent people with dementia from engaging in networks to support one another.

> ### An example of a user-led network of people with dementia: Contribution from the Scottish Dementia Working Group (SDWG)
>
> Someone said to me 'Come along in the car and I'll take you out and I'll bring you a sandwich.' I thought, 'What's happened to me?' People said they would sit me out in the garden as if I were a toy. The attitude of people towards us takes away our confidence. That, in a nutshell, is why the SDWG came about. We came together because

we wanted to speak for ourselves. When we formed in 2002, people with dementia were not expected to speak up – or even to be at meetings where dementia was being discussed.

The SDWG was established as a campaigning group, while bringing people with a diagnosis of dementia together to gain support from each other. The group has a committee of 18 members who vote on key issues. Almost all of the most active members are on the committee. About 40 members regularly attend the group meetings either in Glasgow or in Dundee. The remaining members, about half, either do not or rarely attend meetings. They are kept in touch with the work of the group through minutes of meetings, newsletters and our website. With the Scottish Dementia Strategy now being developed, all members will receive regular bulletins, updating them on the progress of the Strategy and encouraging their participation in contributing their thoughts and comments.

We were able to stress the importance of early diagnosis when two members were invited by NHS Quality Improvement Scotland to serve on a working group about integrated care pathways for people with dementia. We want to see support in place from day one. Our awareness-raising work, speaking to doctors, nurses and social workers in training, has demonstrated that there is nothing more powerful than hearing a person speaking from personal experience. If more people receive an early diagnosis they will have more time to make practical arrangements for their future care and will be better able to build a good quality of life for themselves in the meantime. This is exactly what we have been campaigning for.

When a group comprises a membership of people with a deteriorating condition the issue of sustainability is a particular challenge. The SDWG has been running for almost seven years and has been fortunate that a few key members have remained with the group throughout this time; people whose condition has remained relatively stable. However, during this time many active campaigners have come and gone. We are reliant on a constant input of active new members and without this the group would no doubt go into decline. One thing we are trying to get rid of is the phrase 'dementia sufferer'. We prefer to think positively and concentrate on what we can still do. Dementia is not pleasant, but nor is it a totally negative condition.

We know that our membership is drawn from a small part of the 69,500 people with dementia in Scotland. As such, we are also constantly seeking to expand so that we can become more representative of all people in Scotland with dementia. Work is ongoing in building relationships with minority ethnic communities; the group has recently undertaken partnership work with Deaf Connections; and the use of new technology is being explored so that people in remote communities can participate. Our involvement with the Talking Mats project at Stirling University gave us the chance to think about how people in the later stages of the condition can be helped to express their views.

Independence and autonomy are very important to the group, but being under the umbrella of Alzheimer Scotland has provided the infrastructure for the group both to survive and grow. Nevertheless, the group insists on being able to determine its campaigning priorities and is very protective of its right to speak out about the issues that are important to members, the people who are living with a diagnosis of dementia. For further details see: www.sdwg.org.uk.

Guidance and examples of involving people with dementia: Bamford and Bruce (2000); Cantley, Woodhouse and Smith (2005); Cheston, Bender and Byatt (2000); Care Services Improvement Partnership (2007); Keady *et al.* (2007).

Towards inclusive user involvement

'You can just write off users' views you know – here he is being paranoid; here he is being depressed' (service user quoted in Lewis 2009: 21). While user involvement is so often linked to empowerment and influence there is a need to acknowledge its currently fragile status. Beresford and Croft (2001) note that providers have the capacity to obstruct, tokenise and side-track service users, and delay or fail to implement changes. Where divergence appears between users and providers the legitimacy of user groups can be questioned (Harrison and Mort 1998), the rhetoric of participation may be deployed to legitimate cuts and the withdrawal of services (Baker, Brown and Gwilym 2008). In this chapter it has been argued that practitioners have a vital role to play in the process of strengthening involvement mechanisms. This requires navigating the largely uncritical representations of participation contained in policy and the, at times, self-congratulatory accounts of apparently flawless involvement initiatives to be found in the existing literature. In short, there is a need to embrace a more critical perspective on involvement – but what would this entail?

Participation structures: fundamentally, user involvement is about relations of power – something that is often downplayed in much policy output. It would be a mark of progress if power were openly discussed in participatory initiatives. This would support a more nuanced understanding of how power circulates (Foucault 1977) as users engage with one another and with providers. Such discussions would be particularly relevant to mental health services where an imbalance of power is formalised and authorised. Under these conditions it is unhelpful to speak in general terms of user empowerment without a precise understanding of what this implies. Exposing relations of power may seem threatening to practitioners but it may also help foster a debate on empowering practice; and, given that there is no requirement for participation mechanisms to mirror existing structures in the welfare system, such a discussion may help in further developing less or non-hierarchical user networks that take into account other axes of difference.

Methods and evaluation: there is also a need to better demonstrate whether, and to what extent, participation is working (Campbell 2001). This means looking beyond the specific objectives of individual initiatives to consider the broader and longer-term impact of involvement. For instance, to what extent does involvement build social capital within different communities (Callaghan and Wistow 2008), and in what ways might inclusivity be judged as an outcome of user involvement? A particular challenge lies in trying to map the impact of participation as it evolves over time (Webb 2008). A debate is yet to be had on the most relevant methods to capture the complex and lasting effects of user involvement (Frankham 2009).

The involvement process: at a practical level, greater clarity and openness about the participation process in general and discussion of the barriers that currently prevent this would be helpful. Where involvement fails, is appropriated or diverted there is a need to be able to at least document this without repercussions and engage in an open discussion with all those involved. With regard to inclusivity, moving beyond the category of service user would assist in giving an account of who currently gets involved and of those who do not. If barriers to involvement are due to restrictions of time or funding this should be made clear. It would help to develop a profile of participating users to better understand and map out patterns of inclusion/exclusion and to address the persistent omission of certain groups and communities. Moreover, where different forms of exclusion exist, users and practitioners can work together to develop strategies to tackle these. In this way user involvement can support individuals to talk across difference rather than be silenced by it.

Situated knowledge × inclusive measures + empowering practice + funding/resources × time = effective user involvement.

Conclusion

The key ingredients in a recipe for meaningful participation are not difficult to spell out. This chapter has emphasised the importance of inclusivity, and the relationship between sustainable involvement and the capacity to better reflect the diversity of service users. The discussion has taken account not only of the barriers to participation but also the potential for practice to enhance user involvement. It is clear, though, that some factors are beyond the scope of either practitioners or users to control. Effective involvement is most likely to be co-created; the result of close working between users, practitioners, researchers, provider agencies, policy-makers and other key stakeholders including funding bodies.

For all concerned there is a need to engage in a critical debate over the status of different types of knowledge in health and social care and to agree on the importance of sustainable, inclusive and evaluated involvement systems with measures and indicators to support this. Ultimately, the agenda and future direction of user involvement is to be set collectively by users – it is hoped that, with appropriate support, the diversity of those who use services will be reflected in this process.

References

Baker, S., Brown, B. and Gwilym, H. (2008) 'The rise of the service user: are some service users more equal than others?', *Soundings*, 40: 18.

Bamford, C. and Bruce, E. (2000) 'Defining outcomes of community care: the perspectives of older people with dementia and their carers', *Ageing and Society*, 20: 543–70.

Barker, P. and Rolfe, G. (2004) 'Reframing the nurse's role through a social model approach: a rights-based approach to workers' development', *Journal of Psychiatric and Mental Health Nursing*, 11: 365–73.

Barnes, M. and Bennett, G. (1998) 'Frail bodies, courageous voices: older people influencing community care', *Health and Social Care in the Community*, 6 (2): 102–11.

Bartlett, R. and O'Connor, D. (2007) 'From personhood to citizenship: broadening the lens for dementia practice and research', *Journal of Aging Studies*, 21 (2): 107–18.

Beresford, P. and Campbell, J. (1994) 'Disabled people, service users, user involvement and representation', *Disability and Society*, 9 (3): 315–25.

Beresford, P. and Croft, S. (2001) 'Service users' knowledges and the social construction of social work', *Journal of Social Work*, 1 (3): 295–316.

Bochel, C., Bochel, H., Somerville, P. and Worley, C. (2008) 'Marginalised or enabled voices? "User participation" in policy and practice', *Social Policy and Society*, 7: 201–10.

Braye, S. (2000) 'Participation and involvement in social care: an overview', in H. Kemshall and R. Littlechild (eds) *User involvement and participation in social care: research informing practice*, London: Jessica Kingsley.

Callaghan, G. and Wistow, G. (2008) 'Can the community construct knowledge to shape services in the local state? A case study', *Critical Social Policy*, 28 (2): 165–86.

Campbell, P. (2001) 'The role of users of psychiatric services in service development – influence not power', *Psychiatric Bulletin*, 25: 87–88.

Cantley, C., Woodhouse, J. and Smith, M. (2005) *Listen to us: involving people with dementia in planning and developing services*, Newcastle: Dementia North. Available: www.mentalhealthpromotion.net/resources/listen-to-us.pdf (accessed 4 February 2010).

Care Services Improvement Partnership (2007) *Strengthening the involvement of people with dementia: a resource for implementation*, York: Care Services Improvement Partnership.

Carey, M. (2009) 'Happy shopper? The problem with service user and carer participation', *British Journal of Social Work*, 39: 179–88.

Carr, S. (2004) *Has service user participation made a difference to social care services?* Bristol: Social Care Institute for Excellence/Policy Press.

——(2007) 'Participation, power, conflict and change: Theorizing dynamics of service user participation in the social care system of England and Wales', *Critical Social Policy*, 27 (2): 266–76.

Cheston, R., Bender, M. and Byatt, S. (2000) 'Involving people who have dementia in the evaluation of services: a review', *Journal of Mental Health*, 9 (5): 471–79.

Cook, G. and Klein, B. (2005) 'Involvement of older people in care, service and policy planning', *International Journal of Older People Nursing*, 14 (3a): 43–47.

Davies, P. and River, L. (2006) *Being Taken Seriously: The Polari in Partnership Project – promoting change for older lesbians, gay men and bisexuals*, London: Polari.

Department of Health (2006) *National Health Service Act*, London: HMSO.

——(2007) *The Local Government and Public Involvement in Health Act*, London: HMSO.

Dialog (2007) *The Equality Standard for Local Government*, London: IdeA.

Forbes, J. and Sashidharan, S.P. (1997) 'User involvement in services – incorporation or challenge?', *British Journal of Social Work*, 27: 481–98.

Foucault, M. (1977) *Discipline and punish: the birth of the prison*, London: Penguin.

Frankham, J. (2009) *Partnership research: A review of approaches and challenges in conducting research in partnership with service users*, National Centre for Research Methods. Available: eprints.ncrm.ac.uk/778 (accessed 4 February 2010).

Gilliard, C. and Higgs, P. (1998) 'Older people as users and consumers of healthcare: a third age rhetoric for a fourth age reality?', *Ageing and Society*, 18: 233–48.

Gilliard, J., Means, R., Beattie, A. and Daker-White, G. (2005) 'Dementia care in England and the social model of disability', *Dementia: the international journal of social research and practice*, 4 (4): 571–86.

Gould, N. (2006) 'An inclusive approach to knowledge for mental health social work practice and policy', *British Journal of Social Work*, 36: 106–25.

Harrison, S. and Mort, M. (1998) 'Which champions, which public? Public and user involvement in health care as a technology of legitimation', *Social Policy and Administration*, 32 (1): 60–70.

Keady, J., Williams, S., Hughes-Roberts, J., Quinn, P. and Quinn, M. (2007) '"A changing life": co-constructing a personal theory of awareness and adjustment to the onset of Alzheimer's disease', in M. Nolan, E. Hanson, G. Grant and J. Keady (eds) *User participation in health and social care research: voices, values and evaluation*, Maidenhead: Open University Press.

Lewis, L. (2009) 'Politics of recognition: what can a human rights perspective contribute to understanding users' experiences of involvement in mental health services?', *Social Policy and Society*, 8 (2): 211–14.

McDaid, S. (2009) 'An equality of condition framework for user involvement in mental health policy and planning: evidence from participatory action research', *Disability and Society*, 24 (4): 461–74.

McFarlane, L. (1998) *Diagnosis Homophobic: the experiences of lesbians, gay men and bisexuals in mental health services*, London: PACE.

Nolan, M., Hanson, E., Grant, G., Keady, J. and Lennart, M. (2007a) 'Introduction: what counts as knowledge, whose knowledge counts? Towards authentic participatory enquiry', in M. Nolan, E. Hanson, G. Grant and J. Keady (eds) *User participation in health and social care research: voices, values and evaluation*, Maidenhead: Open University Press.

Nolan, M., Hanson, E., Grant, G., Keady, J. and Lennart, M. (2007b) 'Conclusions: realizing authentic participatory enquiry', in M. Nolan, E. Hanson, G. Grant and J. Keady (eds) *User participation in health and social care research: voices, values and evaluation*, Maidenhead: Open University Press.

Office of Public Sector Information (1967) *The Sexual Offences Act*, London: HMSO.

Pawson, R., Boaz, A., Grayson, L., Long, A. and Barnes, C. (2003) *Knowledge review 3: Types and quality of knowledge in social care*, London: Social Care Institute for Excellence.

Perry, A. and Gilbody, S. (2009) 'User-defined outcomes in mental health: a qualitative study and consensus development exercise', *Journal of Mental Health,* 18 (5): 415–23.

Postle, K. and Beresford, P. (2007) 'Capacity building and the reconception of political participation: a role for social care workers', *British Journal of Social Work*, 37: 143–58.

Postle, K., Wright, P. and Beresford, P. (2005) 'Older people's participation in political activity – making their voices heard: a potential support role for welfare professionals in countering ageism and social exclusion', *Practice*, 17 (3): 173–89.

Smith, G., Bartlett, A. and King, M. (2004) 'Treatments of homosexuality in Britain since the 1950s – an oral history: the experience of patients', *British Medical Journal,* 328: 427–29.

Tait, L. and Lester, H. (2005) 'Encouraging user involvement in mental health services', *Advances in Psychiatric Treatment,* 11: 168–75.

Thompson, N. and Thompson, S. (2001) 'Empowering older people: beyond the care model', *Journal of Social Work*, 1 (1): 61–76.

Ward, R., Vass, A.A., Aggarwal, N., Garfield, C. and Cybyk, B. (2008) 'A different story: exploring patterns of communication in residential dementia care', *Ageing and Society*, 28: 629–51.

Webb, S.A. (2008) 'Modelling service user participation in social care', *Journal of Social Work*, 8 (3): 269–90.

Wintrip, S. (2009) *Not safe for us yet – The experiences and view of older lesbians, gay men and bisexuals using mental health services in London*, London: Polari. Available: www.casweb.org/polari/file-storage/index?folder_id=939673&n_past_days = 99999 (accessed 4 February 2010).

2 Social care approaches

Jill Manthorpe

Key messages

- Social care practitioners and social workers will encounter many older people with mental health problems and work with them to provide good quality social care support, to aid recovery and enhance their choices, independence and well-being.
- The local context of services for older people affects social care and social work activities. Such professionals may work in teams with other health colleagues or may work more closely with other colleagues in housing, peer support or community development settings.
- There is little evidence to underpin social care and work practice but emerging accounts of practice and efforts to understand what works and for whom.

Introduction

In the United Kingdom (UK) local authorities or councils with social services responsibilities possess particular powers and responsibilities. They can arrange, pay for or provide services for adults – among whom are disabled people, people with mental health problems and carers. In some areas, provision for older people with mental health problems is very much a joint activity between local authorities and the NHS. In other areas, the NHS provides primary and secondary services, but local councils commission social care services and their delivery is largely in the hands of private and voluntary organisations. The latter are also the main organisational providers of social care for people who pay for services, typically running home care services, alarm systems and care homes.

Legislation generally refers to community care but the term social care is increasingly employed as a way of describing what local authorities do in terms of commissioning services for eligible people, providing such support themselves, and working with other stakeholders to promote mental health and community well-being. In England and Wales, the bedrock of their responsibilities to individuals remains the *National Assistance Act 1948*. This enables local authorities to provide a range of welfare services to disabled people – providing a safety net of support for many older people and others. It is the only part of William Beveridge's post-Second World War foundations of the welfare state that is still in force (Manthorpe 2009). Ideas about need and disabilities have changed, with growing emphasis on human rights, equalities and citizenship, but the role of the local authority in social care remains fundamental.

Other laws relevant to older people with mental health problems widened local authorities' powers and duties. For instance, the *Mental Health Act 1983* placed duties on local authorities and the NHS to provide after-care for people who have been detained in hospital. The *NHS and Community Care Act 1990* (Department of Health 1990) obliged local authorities to conduct community care assessments or assessments of social need at a time when local authorities were moving from being the main providers of social care (home helps and old people's homes, for example), to purchasers or commissioners of services from the private and voluntary sector (Means, Morbey and Smith 2002).

Many laws in the area of social care and mental health affect adults of all ages who have a range of disabilities or long-term conditions that make caring for themselves difficult, and present risks to their own health or well-being, or those of other people. Laws and guidance also apply to distinct client groups and settings. Such is the current complexity that the law in this area is being considered for major review and consolidation, with the Law Commission (2008) describing it as inadequate, incomprehensible and outdated. One example of this complexity forms the basis of the case study below, where a team is working with a person who has decided to use her social care resource allocation though a Direct Payment. Initially, older people were excluded from the *Community Care (Direct Payments) Act 1996*, which allowed local authorities to make payments to people who are eligible for social care services (sometimes known as a personal or individual budget). Older people are now eligible and local authorities have a duty to provide Direct Payments in certain circumstances (*Health and Social Care Act 2001*). Furthermore, under the revised regulations of the *Health and Social Care Act 2008*, if a person lacks the capacity to consent to Direct Payments, for example a person with severe dementia, a payment can be made to a suitable person to manage the Direct Payment on their behalf. I touch on this below.

For anyone working with social care colleagues, the local context also matters. This is not simply because different geographical areas may have different needs and traditions of provision; it is because local authority social care is part of local government. This is distinct from the NHS and the private sector, and gives rise to advantages and disadvantages. On the positive side, it means that local authorities have discretion over what they spend on social care, as opposed to parks or swimming pools, and may view social care as important to community well-being, or it may mean that there is apparently unhelpful political interference or a seemingly endless need to get political party agreement to get decisions ratified. Elected members may be very keen to support services that meet the needs of their constituents and know much about these needs, or they may have a keen interest in keeping council tax low and distrust professionals. The separation of children's and adults' services, common in most parts of England, may give older people's needs a higher profile, or it may mean that adult services are only a minor element of a local authority's interests.

Team working in a local context is framed by tradition, organisational agreements, political choices, professional preferences and happenstance. There may be patterns of team working that have been generated by enthusiasts for co-location, where primary care and social services share buildings and much more, despite the limited evidence that this leads to better outcomes. Much seems to depend on two elements. In one study of joint working, both social workers and doctors interviewed described weaknesses in their working arrangements with their counterparts in social and health care and attributed them to two factors (Kharicha *et al.* 2005). The first was a fundamental lack of understanding and clarity of each other's roles, responsibilities, pressures and organisational procedures. The second factor was particular local combinations of local policies, structures and organisation. Good relationships between middle managers from different agencies may stem from their shared understanding of management roles and similar experiences of pressures in the public sector. Together they may have the capacity to shape local practices and policies, to some degree.

Key policy drivers

Personalisation is reshaping the delivery of social care in England and is influencing practice more widely in the rest of the UK (see Carr 2008). One element of this is the implementation of personal budgets; these aim to shift control to people eligible for publicly funded social care services by allowing them more choice in the organisation of their allocated resource (budget) for their support. This approach is leading to major cultural changes within local authorities at team, practitioner, and service user and carer levels. It is inevitably affecting relationships with other organisations, professionals and teams.

The theme of personalisation of support in adult social care emerged in policy documents covering health and social care, including *Improving the life choice of disabled people* (Department of Health 2005a), *Independence, Well-being and Choice* (Department of Health 2005b), *Our NHS, our future: NHS next stage review* (Department of Health 2007a) and *Putting People First* (Department of Health 2007b). The pilots of Individual Budgets, now more commonly known as personal budgets, indicated the success of these but also pointed to older people's fear of managing the money (Glendinning *et al*. 2008). The Department of Health has made a further commitment to exploring personal budgets in the NHS for some patients (Department of Health 2009). As the case study shortly outlines, the world of social care provision is being changed as a result, with much agreement among practitioners that people using services will potentially have greater opportunities and greater choices and that care will be more tailored (Manthorpe and Stevens 2009). There are also concerns that the move brings with it risks of individualising social care (Ferguson 2007) and may lead to increased risks of harm for some individuals unless support plans are alert to this (Manthorpe *et al*. forthcoming). Will a local day centre survive, for instance, if a number of people prefer to employ a Personal Assistant instead? Will people be exploited under the new arrangements – services users, family members or social care workers?

While these developments apply to social care provision, other recent policy changes are structural, but locally specific in implementation. Following the introduction of the *NHS and Community Care Act 1990* (Department of Health 1990), for example, the Government re-asserted its commitment to better co-ordinated services, in particular through mechanisms such as the care programme approach and care management (Lester and Glasby 2006) and multi-disciplinary community mental health teams (CMHTs) (Challis *et al*. 2002). These had important implications for local authority mental health services, and the work of their specialist mental health staff, Approved Social Workers. Established as a role with some independence from medical influence, this role was able to access some directly provided local authority services, such as counselling, day care, home care and short-breaks, while providing advocacy for older people undergoing care and treatment in NHS provider units. The advent of integrated Health and Social Care Trusts in some areas and the *Health Act 1999* provided the framework for further partnership working between health and social services and greater expansion of CMHTs. However, the National Audit Office census (National

Audit Office 2007) exposed their variations, for example, in the availability of their support for people with dementia at home:

- Telecare – available to 34 percent of Teams, but insufficiently funded to make it available for 11 percent of Teams and not available to 31 percent of Teams.
- Respite or short breaks – available to 67 percent of Teams, insufficiently funded for 23 percent of Teams and not available to 6 percent of Teams.
- Day care – available to 74 percent of Teams, insufficiently funded for 3 percent of Teams and not available to 19 percent of Teams.

(National Audit Office 2007: Table O)

In spite of these initiatives and positive reports, problems remain. For example, social workers continue to fear domination by the NHS and loss of social care leadership. Brown, Tucker and Domokos (2003) pointed to the continuance of belief, rather than evidence, that such integration will produce better outcomes. They observed that until social services and NHS Trusts develop more efficient and compatible information systems, it is actually hard to evaluate what impact integration is having on older people. Yet, in spite of these factors, a number of political, financial and practical imperatives continue to promote integrated service development, not least to provide service users and carers with easy access to services to prevent problems getting worse.

Partnerships and CMHTs have led to joint management arrangements and the blurring of boundaries between professional roles, in particular between community nursing and social work. For example, nurses are increasingly writing the social circumstances report when a detained patient appeals to a Mental Health Review Tribunal, traditionally the task of social workers, and taking on duties of social support and after-care (Rapaport and Manthorpe 2008). Social workers may be key workers for people with dementia and be able to make referrals to secondary NHS services directly for specialist assessments (Das and Bouman 2008).

One further feature influences team working with older people who have mental health problems: much social care is means tested in the UK, but NHS care and treatment are not. Paying for care is not new but it has a major impact on older people's attitudes to social care services; it often leads to people who have to pay for their own care (self-funders) being excluded from social care support; and it complicates joint NHS and local authority services. Local authority assessments include financial assessments; a task that no other profession seems keen to take on.

Applying principles

About the team

In this chapter I first take two examples related to dementia services, one reflecting work in a local authority that is embracing new ways of working in line with the Department of Health's policy to transform social care. We shall call this place Holby City and, although this is fictional, it rests on events occurring in a variety of local authorities. The second team is situated in the fictional area of Walford (readers will identify misspent evenings watching UK television soaps). Here there is not so great change envisaged and a settled pattern of organisational relationships is evident. The case study, however, is common to both areas and, of course, anonymised.

Case study

Margaret and Bill Myers live in the council house they bought in the 1980s. They are both in their mid-70s. Their daughter Susan lives nearby. Mr Myers retired from his job on the railways 20 years ago, now spending his time round the house and garden, and helping in the local Trade Union Social Club. Other family members are on friendly terms, but generally the couple keep themselves to themselves, apart from the Club.

Susan pops in to her parents every week. One Saturday morning she is surprised to find her mother is still in her dressing gown and very upset. Mrs Myers says that they have had a dreadful night as her husband thinks that Club members are ganging up on him. He has been worried about this for weeks but things have come to a head. He has fallen asleep, at last, on the sofa.

Susan makes a cup of tea and suggests that her mother goes for a nap or has a bath while she tidies up. She herself has thought her father increasingly out of sorts recently but did not realise his distress. The family spend a subdued weekend, with Susan resolving to call her parents' general practitioner (GP) on Monday.

Three months later, a lot has happened. Mr Myers has been to his GP, who has conducted various tests and assessments, making an appointment for him to go to a memory assessment service. Mrs Myers became exhausted with lack of sleep and her GP has suggested that she tries a course of sleeping tablets, for the time being. Susan is calling on her parents more regularly and has been further concerned that several bills are unpaid and that her mother seems not so able to cope now her father is still under the weather. She had not realised how much of the housework and shopping he must have been doing.

Three months later, Mr Myers has been to the memory clinic, had various tests and spent time with the doctor there. He has been told that he has Alzheimer's disease, that the clinic staff will offer him support and that if drugs seem to be suitable, then they will be available. Mrs Myers has also seen someone at the clinic who has given her details of the local carers' group. Mr Myers resigned from the Social Club, now spending most of his time sitting in front of the television. Mrs Myers is increasingly tearful and the house is becoming unkempt. Susan is worried about things and shocked to hear her parents arguing and shouting at each other.

Assessment approaches

Here, I focus on what happens in relation to the Myers family in respect of social care services. Unlike the NHS and its first port of call with the GP, there are several ways in which the family may get in touch with local authority social services, or they may not for some time, or even never. But let us consider what might happen in Holby.

At the memory assessment service, Mr Myers's case was allocated to a key worker (Ellen Smith) who keeps in contact with the family. While based in the memory assessment service, this key worker post is funded by both the local Primary Care Trust and the local social services department. Ellen is social work qualified, but many of the people she talks to think she is a nurse or doctor. Susan phones Ellen about the possibility of getting a home help and describes what is happening. Ellen suggests that they meet with her parents, in their home, to discuss what they would like and to consider some options. Ellen, in effect, is beginning to carry out an assessment of Mr Myers and Mrs Myers, asking their permission to contact their GP for further information and collecting details of their income and savings. She had earlier suggested that they claim certain income maintenance and disability benefits, and she checks how this went. Following this meeting – in which the family talks about wanting some company for Mr Myers, perhaps to take him to the Social Club, and some ways they might be helped so that their home stays clean and comfortable – a support plan is sketched out. The family meet with Ellen to discuss the ways to put this plan into action, and Ellen suggests that the family might like to manage the budget and so bring in support at the times when it is needed. One element that Susan is keen on is using the budget to pay the rental charges for an alarm system that her parents can use to call for help if they are in trouble.

The elements of this assessment are clear to the family. The support plan is one that they have discussed and built up. They feel that nothing precipitous is happening; that Mr Myers will not be with continual strangers; that Mrs Myers will not be too anxious because Susan is involved. This has been an assessment under the *NHS and Community Care Act 1990*, but, to the family, it has been a way of getting things to seem a bit more normal and back on track.

How has this seamless and efficient process come about? Behind it lie protocols and agreements within and between statutory agencies (NHS and local government). Significantly more multidisciplinary assessments are being undertaken following the introduction of the Single Assessment Process (SAP) in England, particularly by occupational therapists and secondary health care teams. Cognitive impairment is a significant predictor of multidisciplinary assessment (Sutcliffe *et al.* 2008). The SAP enabled Ellen to build on information already collected and did not require the family to repeat their details and story. The occupational therapist talked with Ellen about the possible alarm systems and other aids. Moving to complete the community care assessment, Ellen was able to determine eligibility (moderate), to estimate the resources available from local government, to develop a support plan, and to get details on what the family will have to contribute. She had access to systems to set up the assistive technology (the alarm system and eventually other aids). She was able to concentrate on the possible different needs and perspectives of the family, and the potential for these to change. The family think Ellen is helpful and are not bothered about how her role relates to those of other members of the wider teams involved; they presume that she is talking to them.

Matters such as planning were addressed in some of Mr Myers's early discussions with the clinical psychologist, as documented in the electronic notes (with the SAP) that Ellen consulted. The family received general leaflets about the *Mental Capacity Act 2005* and other information, and Susan has been thinking about discussing Lasting Power of Attorney with her parents. She wants to get some of the more practical things sorted before this, particularly the state of the home. Ellen reassures her that if the family does not want to organise support themselves, then the local authority will do this, or put them in touch with a local independent brokerage service, experienced in managing Direct Payments.

A year later, much has changed. Mr Myers is not well and his ability to manage everyday activities is much worse. Mrs Myers became increasingly anxious but a course of antidepressants from her GP seems to be working and she has talked to someone at the local carers' group. Ellen has helped the family revise the support plan, and in doing this she has carried out a carer's assessment for both Mrs Myers and Susan, to help them think about their own needs and wishes. Her parents' decline saddens Susan but the support package is working out as well as it could. Her parents are employing the daughter of a friend to provide 14 hours' housework and some personal care each week (more when Susan is away); the alarm system is reassuring (to Susan) and her parents did use it when the keys got lost. A local employment agency has found a retired man to talk about railways and so on with Mr Myers, three afternoons a week. All this is covered by the support plan (a first attempt to employ a local cleaner failed miserably) and the brokerage service does the necessary paperwork. Mr Myers drew up a Lasting Power of Attorney document, also putting all the household bills and bank accounts in all the family names. When Ellen moves on, the new key worker keeps in touch and has already reviewed the support plan.

If this seems too good to be true, we can consider the case of the family as residents of Walford. Here the memory assessment service runs within a non-integrated organisational structure; not a problem necessarily, but there are formalities that are different and the processes of referral and assessments run in parallel. The memory service refers the family back to the GP once the diagnosis is made and the GP writes to offer support but somehow this gets lost in the general distress of the diagnosis. Susan hears how social services are under pressure and when she drops into the local social services office it is full and depressing. The local voluntary group she calls always seems to have the answerphone on. Mrs Myers is worried that officials will take her husband into an old people's home, where she feels he will be neglected, and pleads with Susan not to call in the social workers. Susan struggles to support her parents but the level of their arguments worries her increasingly. If the words 'care team' were mentioned to Susan, she wouldn't know whether to laugh or cry. One Sunday she calls round to find her mother on the floor, having fallen apparently, and her father very agitated. Her mother is taken to hospital and when the out-of-hours GP comes round to see her father, the GP suggests that her father, too, is admitted for assessment, in his best interests.

The outcomes are not surprising. Mrs Myers's fracture takes a while to heal and Mr Myers is moved from the assessment ward to a care home. A social worker spends some time negotiating this and seems to work a lot around a mystifying fax (Mr Myers's needs are seen as critical). In the care home Mr Myers's mobility takes a turn for the worse, he becomes incontinent and the care workers seek medication to help them cope with his aggressive behaviour. The local authority (social services) pays for his care home place and this is reviewed every year, but not in great depth. Just after one year in the care home Mr Myers dies. Mrs Myers, however, did return home and a reablement home care package was briefly put in place. Susan struggles to support her mother, calling on her GP increasingly frequently. There are many care teams that the family have come across at this stage: the team of staff at the care home; the reablement team; the hospital teams; the primary care team; and so forth. However, often Susan feels that she is on her own ....

The fax that Susan hears about is the Fair Access to Care System (FACS) that the social services uses to determine eligibility for publicly funded social care. This provides local government with guidance about the ways they should review, revise and use their eligibility criteria for access to adult care services in order to achieve greater equity in social care services to local people (Charles and Manthorpe 2009). The early aspirations for eligibility criteria were that:

> Authorities should have clear rules about who can get help – for instance, in what sorts of circumstances someone would get help with dressing or washing at home. These rules (usually known as eligibility criteria) should mean that everyone in that area gets treated fairly ... there must be national standards so that we can

avoid some people not getting the level of quality of service that Parliament has said should be available everywhere ...

(Department of Health 1998: paragraph 1.4)

The social worker in Walford was thinking of eligibility criteria continually, whereas in Holby, the FACS system was similar but less overtly operated. All practitioners in social services operate under financial constraints. FACS is one way to ration resources, and its limits give rise to continual calls for social care funding to be better resourced (Wanless 2006), most recently in the *National Dementia Strategy* in England (Department of Health 2009).

Cases in context

One key part of this jigsaw of social and health care services is the organisational context of social care services, and the possible difficulties where specialist practitioners are organisationally or professionally isolated from broader social care services. Where this is the case, the question arises of the extent to which an almost exclusive focus on dementia (or visual impairment, or depression, or ethnicity, or learning disability and so on) in some areas of social care practice mirrors medical perspectives that isolate specific traits. These approaches may reflect the use of individualised definitions of disability that emphasise a medically defined condition at the expense of identifying the social and environmental impacts of disability related to dementia; such issues are explored further in Chapters 7, 8 and 9 of this book. Debates about the social care of older people with dementia are part of wider considerations about the social care of older people and of people with disabilities in general. Combinations of disabilities are increasingly likely among older people.

There is variation in assessment and provision throughout the social care system for people with dementia, and all other disabilities and needs. Some may be attributable to varying levels of expertise between specialists and non-specialists, but others reflect differences arising from the availability of local resources, which in turn influence the different levels of eligibility criteria. Weiner *et al.* (2002: 437) observed that such inequity was endemic in their study of general social care provision.

In England the *National Dementia Strategy* (Department of Health 2009) is partly intended to reform the unpredictability and inadequacy currently characterising social care provision where much depends on local patterns of provision and care markets, commitments to expenditure and resources, and rationing systems, such as FACS. It may be that the starting point is not to use dementia always as the defining characteristic but to spread expertise equitably within social care services. If this were so then the starting point would be that:

- some older people have social care needs related to their dementia (such as Mr Myers's needs for company, home care and stimulation); and
- might also have other social care needs not related to dementia but which might also be disabling (such as Mrs Myers's need for help in the home and her need for reassurances); and
- have needs arising as much (and possibly more) from the disabling impact of the social environment, as from a medically defined impairment (such as being unable to summon help); and

- access to services that respond to these needs is provided in the context of the disproportionate power of the social and health care sectors (such as the lack of skilled support in and resources of the care home to promote continence and mobility, to manage behaviour that challenges, and so on).

For the Myers family, Mr Myers's needs arise from a number of causes and stressors, not just his dementia. While in Holby these are being responded to, in Walford they are narrowly defined. Social care support should be explicitly orientated towards maintaining independence and quality of life (Department of Health 2006), goals which are already implicit in much specialist assessment practice. This requires that practitioners should explore the types of social care needs arising from dementia, but that this might be more timely and more effective if undertaken earlier and in partnership, as needs are often gradual in onset and social in origin.

The two scenarios present different ways forward for strategic and joint commissioners across health and social care services. In some areas, intensive care management provided by an old age mental health service may be an attractive option, although health staff's adoption of a care management role requires them to be good at making arrangements about information sharing, giving sufficient time to provide the necessary careful assessments of needs, undertaking liaison with a wide range of other agencies, and keeping in close and regular contact with the older person and their care network (Tucker *et al.* 2008). Rather than expect nurses to be social workers, it may be that team working can be more a complementary than a substitution process.

In other areas, a rational system or clinical care pathway might be in place, but the elements or pieces depend on developing understanding and clarity about each other's roles, agreements about responsibilities, capacity to manage wider pressures and organisational procedures that focus on the needs of the people with mental health problems concerned and their supporters. Local combinations of policies, structures and organisation can either assist in care that is person-centred or make it difficult. Leadership is central, of course, with skilled social care leaders knowing how their own roles interweave with those of leaders within more hierarchical organisations and professions.

The case scenario of Mr Myers in this chapter draws attention to the many possible teams involved when social care services are involved. Any discussion of team working, care or case management is affected by the differing levels of intensity with which it is delivered. People using services and their carers may value the support and attention that they receive as a result of key working or care/case management. Others may, however, think it intrusive. Nevertheless, whatever personal and organisational authority practitioners command, much depends on whether they are able to influence the work of a wide range of staff in other commissioning and provider agencies, and further social networks. Care/case managers, key workers or navigators, or dementia advisers on their own, cannot compensate for over-fragmented health and social care services. Safety nets of the voluntary sector, advocates or family carers are not always able to patch up threadbare services or to challenge existing ways of doing things. In this case scenario, we have observed that social care teams are not a reality for many people. Some carers, like Susan, are the main provider or manager of care, and the team that she assembles around her needs to be effective. One new commitment from public sector social care is to work with the grain of informal care, rather than to work against it. Knowledge of communities and widely defined social care support has to be part of the network of support for people with dementia and other needs.

Social care services for people with depression

Older people in the main have good mental health, but they are more prone to risk factors for later life depression, including physical disability, pain and illness and its effect on daily living, as well as social isolation and loneliness, often the result of bereavement (Age Concern and the Mental Health Foundation 2007). It has long been recognised that depression is the most common mental disorder in older people (Livingston *et al.* 1990) and for many individuals this has a profound impact on their quality of life and well-being. Interdisciplinary practice can help older people and their carers, and it can also be a means whereby practitioners themselves may feel supported.

In a third case scenario, I consider the case of an older woman whose distant family interpret their mother's circumstances as requiring social care support.

Mrs Grove is experiencing panic attacks that leave her frightened and tearful for reasons about which she is not clear. They have been growing in intensity since she was moved out of her home temporarily when there was risk of flooding in the street. She is frightened of being seen as mad, and frightened that she will lose her home. Her daughter who lives in another city thinks her mother may have some sort of heart problem as she complains about her heart racing and feeling sweaty. Ms Grove decides that her mother needs more help round the house, and that home care is necessary. She contacts the local authority and asks for Mrs Grove to be assessed for home care. The social worker assigned to conduct an assessment is faced with asking whether it matters why Mrs Grove is having what sound like panic attacks, or wheter she should focus on helping her to deal with them, perhaps through some help round the home, that might gently encourage her to go out and regain her usual activities. While not clinically qualified, the experience of this social worker is considerable in working with older people with depression, such is the high prevalence of depression among social care users. At initial assessment the social worker will ask Mrs Grove if she has other symptoms that to her might be suggesting depression (for example, loss of energy, appetite, interest, or weight; sleeplessness; multiple aches and pains).

If Mrs Grove's answers are negative then reassurance that panic attacks always come to an end may be appropriate, along with supportive counselling until they do, and medication to control physical symptoms (if necessary and safe). The social worker will likely suggest that Mrs Grove go for a check-up with her GP, encouraging her to do this. She keeps in touch with Ms Grove while respecting Mrs Grove's possible desires to keep some matters private.

Underlying this social worker's practice are her own training and experience of working with older people and her mutually informative contacts with other local professionals. She knows the most salient features of anxiety and depression, and their overlap, and that anxiety is typified by feelings of worry, fearfulness, distress, or panic that seem out of proportion or inexplicable. She is also aware that depression can have all of those feelings, plus sadness, tearfulness, loss of confidence, a feeling of worthlessness and loss of appetite. More recently, her participation in local training sessions about the recognition of early dementia has confirmed her experience that complaints about poor memory and concentration may be features of late-life depression.

Many social workers working with older people will have a low threshold for seeking expert advice and involvement, but others will see responding to anxiety symptoms as part of their task. It is not an easy task, because anxiety can take a range of forms – it can exist as a problem in its own right but also as a symptom of other disorders, and it is very individual in nature, as Georgina Charlesworth and Janet Carter further describe in Chapter 4 of this book. If a social worker is part of a CMHT then access to support should be easier, while for others there will be a pattern or procedure (written down or otherwise) of how social workers seek help from their colleagues in community mental health nursing, general practice, psychology or old age psychiatry.

Mrs Grove may well respond to brief cognitive behaviour therapy from a suitably trained therapist accessed through primary care, but she may need medical assessment, even if she has initially refused, because she may have underlying mental health problems with an overlay of anxiety. It is here that the social worker can work with Mrs Grove and her daughter to encourage a visit to the GP, who may call on an old age psychiatrist if the diagnosis is unclear. Particularly worrying features that would prompt such a call are generalised anxiety (about everything), paranoid ideas, obsessions, memory loss and confusion. As noted earlier, it has been established that social workers may have the expertise and experience to make appropriate referrals directly to secondary mental health services, in relation to cases involving both dementia and depression (Manthorpe and Iliffe 2005, Das and Bouman 2008).

In the interim, the social worker may arrange some home care support for Mrs Grove, seeing this as part of reablement or a move to recovery. In the contract with the home care provider, she will discuss the care plan agreed with Mrs Grove, noting that the home care worker should get in touch with the social worker if Mrs Grove appears to be in greater distress or her behaviour is changing for the worse. The social worker also notes that in the event of further threats of flooding, then Mrs Grove should be contacted immediately by the emergency services and establishes that she will have some priority in these circumstances. She gives Mrs Grove information about the local flood prevention scheme and offers her details about the local Age Concern group that offers an insurance service. Part of the support plan set up around the short term home care service is to help Mrs Grove with establishing some sense of order about practicalities in the home, should flooding reoccur as a risk.

Conclusion

Depression is the commonest mental health problem in later life, and social workers are part of the helping and treatment network. They are resources in themselves, and when working with colleagues with other skills and experiences, they are able to provide short- and long-term support. Above all, they may have access to community and informal resources with which other colleagues are less familiar. Such skills are needed when working with people who have dementia and depression and their carers, both at the start of the dementia or disability trajectory and when supporting people at the end of their lives. While the word 'holistic' is rarely used to describe social care and social work practice, it may be highly applicable to the social model of disability and illness that social workers and social care practitioners adopt when working with people who have mental health problems in later life, as the case examples in this chapter have illustrated.

References

Age Concern and the Mental Health Foundation (2007) *Improving services and support for older people with mental health problems. The second report from the UK inquiry into mental health and well-being in later life,*

London: Age Concern and the Mental Health Foundation. Available: www.mhilli.org/documents/Inquiryfinalreport-fullreport.pdf (accessed 4 February 2010).

Brown, L., Tucker, C. and Domokos, T. (2003) 'Evaluating the impact of integrated health and social care teams on older people living in the community', *Health and Social Care in the Community*, 11(2): 85–94.

Carr, S. (2008) *Personalisation: a rough guide*, London, SCIE. Available: www.scie.org.uk (accessed 4 February 2010).

Challis, D., von Abendorff, R., Brown, P., Chesterman, J. and Hughes, J. (2002) 'Care management, dementia and specialist mental health services: an evaluation', *International Journal of Geriatric Psychiatry*, 17: 315–25.

Charles, N. and Manthorpe, J. (2009) 'An exploratory qualitative study of equity and the social care needs of visually impaired older people in England', *British Journal of Visual Impairment*, 27 (2): 97–109.

Das, S. and Bouman, P. (2008) 'Direct referrals from social services to community teams for older people with mental illness', *Psychiatric Bulletin*, 32: 164–65.

Department of Health (1990) *NHS and Community Care Act*, London: HMSO.

——(1998) *Modernising Social Services: promoting independence, improving protection, raising standards*, London: The Stationery Office. Cm 4169.

——(2005a) *Improving the life choice of disabled people*, London: Department of Health.

——(2005b) *Independence, Well-being and Choice: Our Vision for the Future of Social Care for Adults in England*, London: Department of Health.

——(2006) *Our Health, Our Care, Our Say*, London: Department of Health.

——(2007a) *Our NHS, our future: NHS next stage review*, London: Department of Health.

——(2007b) *Putting People First*, London: Department of Health.

——(2009) *Living well with dementia, a National Dementia Strategy*, London: Department of Health.

Ferguson, I. (2007) 'Increasing User Choice or Privatizing Risk? The Antinomies of Personalization', *British Journal of Social Work*, 37(3): 387–403.

Glendinning, C., Challis, D., Fernandez, J.L., Jacobs, S., Jones, K., Knapp, M., Manthorpe, J., Moran, N., Netten, A., Stevens, M. and Wilberforce, M. (2008) *The evaluation of the individual budget pilots*, York: Social Policy Research Unit, University of York. Available: www.york.ac.uk (accessed 4 February 2010).

Kharicha, K., Iliffe, S., Levin, E., Davey, B. and Fleming, C. (2005) 'Tearing down the Berlin Wall: Social workers' perspectives on joint working with general practice', *Family Practice*, 22 (4): 399–405.

Law Commission (2008) *Adult social care; scooping report*, London: Law Commission.

Lester, H. and Glasby, J. (2006) *Mental Health: Policy and Practice*, London: Palgrave Macmillan.

Livingston, G., Hawkins, A., Graham, N., Blizard, B. and Mann, A. (1990) 'The Gospel Oak Study: Prevalence rates of dementia, depression and activity limitation among elderly residents in Inner London', *Psychological Medicine*, 20: 137–46.

Manthorpe, J. (2009) 'Law and policy in older people's mental health policy and practice', in T. Williamson (ed.) *Older people's mental health today: a handbook*, Brighton: Pavilion.

Manthorpe, J. and Iliffe, S. (2005) 'Timely responses to dementia: exploring the social work role', *Journal of Social Work*, 5: 191–203.

Manthorpe, J. and Stevens, M. (2009) 'Increasing Care Options in the Countryside: Developing an Understanding of the Potential Impact of Personalization for Social Work with Rural Older People', *British Journal of Social Work*, Advance Access published on 27 March 2009; doi:10.1093/bjsw/bcp038.

Manthorpe, J., Stevens, M., Rapaport, J., Challis, D., Jacobs, S., Netten, A., Knapp, M., Wilberforce, M. and Glendinning, C. (forthcoming) 'Individual budgets and adult safeguarding: parallel or converging tracks? Further findings from the evaluation of the individual budget pilots', *Journal of Social Work*.

Means, R., Morbey, H. and Smith, R. (2002) *From Community Care to Market Care: The Development of Welfare Services for Older People*, Bristol: Policy Press.

National Audit Office (2007) *Improving services and support for people with dementia*, London: The Stationery Office.

Rapaport, J. and Manthorpe, J. (2008) 'Mental Capacity Act and Mental Health Act', *Journal of Integrated Care*, 16 (4): 22–29.

Sutcliffe, C., Hughes, J., Abendstern, M., Clarkson, P. and Challis, D. (2008) 'Developing multi-disciplinary assessment – exploring the evidence from a social care perspective', *International Journal of Geriatric Psychiatry*, 23 (12): 1297–305.

Tucker, S., Hughes, J., Sutcliffe, C. and Challis, D. (2008) 'Care management for older people with mental health problems: from evidence to practice', *Australian Health Review: a publication of the Australian Hospital Association*, 32 (2): 210–22.

Wanless, D. (2006) *Securing Good Care for Older People*, London: King's Fund.

Weiner, K., Stewart, K., Hughes, J., Challis, D. and Darton, R. (2002) 'Care management arrangements for older people in England: key areas of variation in a national study', *Ageing and Society*, 22 (4): 419–39.

3 Mental health promotion in later life

Ann Crosland and Annie Wallace

Key messages

- Later life can bring with it particular vulnerabilities to a range of mental health problems such as anxiety and depression.
- As the number of older people increases, so too does the need to promote positive mental health and reduce the risk of mental health problems developing.
- Maintaining relationships with others, participation in meaningful activity, physical health issues, discrimination and poverty all have an impact on mental health in later life.
- Interventions to promote positive mental health need to be considered at a structural, community and individual level to be effective.
- Mental health promotion should be integral to all health improvement activities in later life.

Introduction

The promotion of positive mental health in older people has long been a neglected area in research, policy and practice. This neglect appears to be rooted in assumptions about deteriorating mental health being a normal part of the process of ageing and that mental ill health in older people is different to that in the rest of the population. This is illustrated by the way in which mental health services for older people in the United Kingdom (UK) are separated from those for people of working age; for instance, the former tend to focus on the care and treatment of organic brain diseases whilst the latter look at a much wider spectrum of problems. There is little evidence to support these assumptions, and more recent research indicates that mental ill health and mental health problems in later life are complex and varied, but that much more could be done to promote positive mental health and to intervene earlier to prevent mental health problems in older people (Age Concern and the Mental Health Foundation 2006).

Mental health is important as it has a strong influence on a person's motivation, capacity and opportunities to make health choices (Freidli *et al.* 2007). It also helps protect against a range of mental health issues, including mental illness. Recent research suggests that the scale of mental health problems in older people has been greatly underestimated, with common mental health problems such as depression affecting up to 16 percent of the general population of older people at any one time (Cole and Dendukuri 2004); but this is only part of the picture. As the number of people in older age groups increases, so too does the range of experiences and mental health issues they may face.

Not only do pre-existing mental health problems such as depression, anxiety, schizophrenia or bi-polar disorder span into later life, but also new problems, which can predispose older people to mental health issues, can present themselves for the first time. Physical decline, the onset of chronic ill health, social isolation and bereavement are all life experiences that are not exclusive to, but increase in, later years, and magnify the risk of developing mental health problems. They also all provide opportunities for early intervention to prepare people for coping with difficult issues. However, mental health promotion is about more than providing advice and coping strategies to prevent the onset of new problems or exacerbation of pre-existing ones at an individual level; it is also about looking at what can be done within organisations and across communities to tackle wider social determinants of mental health. Indeed, it is at this level that the greatest impact can be achieved in promoting mental health in older people.

This chapter seeks to explore meanings, principles and models of mental health promotion and how these may apply to people in later life by drawing on examples of community-based mental health promotion projects carried out in the north-east of England.

Defining mental health and mental health promotion

Any attempts to promote positive mental health have to work to a clear definition; however, this cannot be seen in isolation from health in general as mental health is an essential component of an individual's overall health and well-being (Nurse 2009). A useful starting point in finding a working definition is to consider the World Health Organization's (WHO) definition of health in general and mental health in particular:

> To reach a state of complete physical, mental and social well-being, an individual or group must be able to identify and realize aspirations to satisfy needs and to change or cope with the environment. Health is therefore seen as a resource for everyday life, not the objective of living; health is a positive concept emphasising social and personal resources as well as physical capabilities.
>
> (World Health Organization 1986: 1)

Mental health is defined as an ability to cope with life's stresses and make a contribution to our communities:

> ... a state of well-being in which the individual realises his or her own abilities, can cope with normal stresses of life, can work productively and fruitfully and is able to make a contribution to his or her own community.
>
> (World Health Organization 2007: 1)

It is clear that health is about more than the mere absence of disease or illness and must take account of the wider social context within which people live their lives. To this end the WHO definitions are useful in making us think more widely. However, whilst they may provide an ideal to which we all may aspire, they are also virtually unattainable for the majority of people, especially for those who are ill-prepared for coping with stresses or who live in challenging circumstances. They also imply that those living with a long-term condition or mental illness cannot achieve positive mental health.

An alternative and potentially more useful approach to defining mental health is to look at the attributes, values or functions that positive mental health might bring. Alexander (2002) offers the following list:

- Resilience.
- Self-worth, self-value.
- Recognising others' worth.
- A sense of right and wrong.
- Good relationships.
- Playing, learning, contributing.
- Coping strategies that work and are not damaging to self or others.
- Comfortable with own company.
- Optimism.
- Feeling able to have an impact on the world.
- Sense of what is important in life.

The assumption here is that not all of these need to be present for a person to experience positive mental health, but that it offers a menu from which people can draw to improve their sense of well-being regardless of their situation and whether or not they have a recognised mental illness or other mental health problem. It is this definition that underpins the approaches proposed for mental health promotion in later life throughout the remainder of this chapter.

Mental health promotion (improvement) in later life

Since the 1990s a number of attempts have been made to develop models for mental health improvement, to aid understanding and to provide a framework for intervention. There are a number of commonly used models of mental health promotion (often termed mental health improvement) that have relevance in later life and that offer ideas of how improvement can be achieved. Some look at positive and negative influences on mental health, for example McDonald and O'Hara (1998) identify a set of five positive influences on an individual's mental health and well-being: environmental quality, self-esteem, emotional processing, self-management skills and social inclusion. All elements are influential at micro, meso and macro levels. While these consider wider influences on mental health, their primary focus remains on the individual within society.

Perhaps the most useful model is adopted by the Department of Health (2001a), as this not only focuses on the need to look at what should be done for individuals but also offers a framework that considers individuals within the wider communities in which they live as well as the structural issues that may impact upon the choices and options available to them. Here, mental health improvement is an issue that needs to be addressed at an individual, community and structural level, and so seeks to strengthen individuals and communities and to reduce structural barriers in the following ways:

- Strengthening individuals by increasing emotional resilience, promoting self-esteem, life and coping skills, improving parenting, helping individuals manage stress, and promoting good communication skills.

- Strengthening communities by promoting social inclusion and participation, improving environments, increasing access to and improving services, improving organisational settings such as schools and workplaces.
- Lowering structural barriers through reducing discrimination, increasing access to education, meaningful employment and housing.

Not all of these will be achieved in any one activity, but any mental health promotion activity should aim to consider each of these three domains.

Increasingly, mental health improvement, or indeed any health improvement activity, can be seen to have a political dimension. For example, WHO has considered mental health promotion as a human rights issue and suggests not only that mental health is fundamental to quality of life of individuals but that: 'Mental health promotion increases the quality of life and well-being of the whole population' (World Health Organization 2005: 1).

One particularly important construct here that appears to underpin all of these models to a greater or lesser extent is that of social capital, as it offers approaches to building communities such that resilience is located across communities (in this sense community could be an organisation or a community of interest, and not simply a location), and not just within individuals:

> On the one hand, millions of dollars are committed to alleviating ill-health through individual intervention meanwhile we ignore what our everyday experience tells us (i.e. the way we organise our society, the extent to which we encourage interaction among the citizenry and the degree to which we trust and associate with each other in caring communities is probably the most important determinant of our health).
>
> (Lomas 1998)

According to Cooper *et al.* (1999), social capital refers to a set of resources within communities, usually a variant on the following categories:

- Social resources, e.g. informal arrangements between neighbours.
- Collective resources, e.g. self-help groups, credit unions, community safety schemes.
- Economic resources, e.g. levels of unemployment, access to green open spaces.
- Cultural resources, e.g. libraries, art centres, schools.

It embodies notions of respect, feeling safe and valuing the visual environment, together with structural issues like access to services and economic development. Social capital includes notions of how people feel about their neighbourhood and is a useful concept within a broad health promotion framework, as it addresses a number of health issues in an holistic way and goes some way toward moving mental health promotion from an individualised concept to something that occurs within communities and organisations.

Why mental health improvement and older people?

If health is to be described in holistic terms, then interventions should routinely address the determinants of mental health as they do those of physical health. Older people have particular mental health improvement needs based on the vulnerabilities older age brings. A report by the Social Exclusion Unit (2006) highlights some major risk factors for the development of mental health problems in later life. These include social isolation, chronic physical illness, poverty and lack of social participation. The last of these, i.e. social participation, is further influenced by fear of crime, lack of access to transport, experiences of age discrimination, lack of access to social activities, and organisations failing to recognise diversity.

Whilst mental ill health or mental health problems are not an inevitable part of ageing, a number of changes that occur in later life can increase an older person's vulnerability to a range of common mental health issues. Those changes include bereavement, caring responsibilities, retirement, isolation and chronic ill health amongst others, all of which point to a need to offer more support and advice to help people prepare for change and increase their resilience and coping skills. The clinical context chapters in Part 2 of this book further develop some of these concerns.

Interventions to improve mental health in later life

In general, health improvement interventions follow the models already described, at a structural level to address the determinants of health, at a community level to address issues of social capital, or at the level of the individual to boost resilience or skill. However, the evidence base for many interventions remains weak (Freidli *et al.* 2007).

In recent years, mental health promotion has received more attention in general, but much of this work has been focused on the needs of young people and those of working age, and thus fails to address the specific needs of older people. Health improvement departments have sought to intervene early at both a community and structural level through the development of activities in settings where people carry out their day-to-day activities and where change can be addressed at all three levels, i.e. individual, community and structural. However, the settings used have tended to be those accessed by children, young people or adults of working age such as schools, colleges and workplaces. Within these settings changes to policies and practice have been sought at the same time as individuals have been encouraged to make lifestyle changes and improve their and their families' health. At this time specific lifestyle issues are also addressed, such as tobacco or healthy-eating initiatives, to influence the activities and lifestyles of individuals and communities. Furthermore, older people tend not to access large organisations but are more community based, and therefore more difficult to reach using these approaches. Other difficulties arise from the focus on specific topics, which fail to address multiple needs or the health of the whole person. This can result in a loss of a wide range of opportunities for the promotion of mental health issues.

An alternative approach to mental health improvement in older people would be to take a life course approach and target interventions on older people. This is the approach adopted by many voluntary and third sector organisations. There are many lessons to be learned from the health improvement initiatives that they have developed over the years, as well as from their experiences of implementing the evidence-based conclusions. A UK inquiry into mental health and well-being published by Age Concern and the Mental Health Foundation (2006) summarises much of this work, and highlights five key areas that have an important impact on mental health in later life, which should be considered in developing interventions for mental health improvement; these are: maintaining relationships; participation in meaningful activity; physical health; discrimination; and poverty. Each of these can be addressed at a structural, community or individual level, and provide a useful starting point for considering interventions to improve the mental health of older people. The remainder of this chapter will look at each of these five areas in turn to identify the nature of the potential problems they pose for older people, and case studies of community-based interventions that have been successfully used to address them in the north-east of England.

Maintaining social relationships

It is estimated that 1 million older people are living in social isolation and that this number will increase steadily as we see an increasingly ageing population in the UK (Age Concern and the Mental Health Foundation 2006). The most isolated are those over 75, those whose partners have died and those living alone. There are also particular issues for some ethnic communities, gay, lesbian and bisexual older people (as also discussed by Richard Ward and his colleagues in Chapter 1 of this book), and those living in rural and therefore geographically isolated communities.

Older people's vulnerability to social isolation can be increased because:

- Transport may be unsuitable, or in some rural communities unavailable, particularly for those with a disability.
- Reduced income can lead to an inability to afford social activities or the transport to get to them.
- Social networks can become reduced when work is no longer a feature of the daily routine.
- Networks diminish as people get older and family and friends die.
- Fear of crime may lead to reluctance to go out, particularly after dark.
- Disability and declining physical health can reduce social activities.

In recent years a range of initiatives has been developed to address the issue of social isolation in later life, including:

- Activity-based programmes like carpet bowls and tea dances designed to attract older participants to improve physical health but also to build social networks.
- Intergenerational projects that aim to break down barriers across generations, to bring people together in mutually beneficial activities. Older people's forums also exist in many local authority areas to give older people a voice in shaping services.
- Pets as companions: having a pet is associated with improved mental health (McNicholas *et al.* 2005).
- Social prescribing initiatives that can be used to build social networks where an older person may be supported to attend a local group or educational activity as part of their treatment.
- The use of information technology as a mechanism for connecting people.

The following case study focuses on a befriending project aimed at reducing social isolation by engaging older people in social activity or one-to-one home befriending.

Case study 1: The Good Companions Project

The Good Companions Project was carried out by Age Concern Gateshead (2004), although a similar approach runs across many areas of the country.

The basic aim of the project was to reduce social isolation by matching volunteer visitors with isolated older people using a range of methods. Socially isolated people were defined as those without existing social networks because of disability, bereavement or geographical disadvantage. The target population was therefore the older end of the ageing population who found getting out and about particularly challenging. The project employed one full-time and one part-time member of staff plus 55 volunteers, and was funded by Tyne and Wear Health Action Zone.

The project had four main elements:

1 A volunteer befriending service.
2 A telephone befriending service.
3 Bereavement support.
4 Setting up social groups.

The befriending service was based on the premise that this would: promote the use of local services and facilities; create new social links; develop wider social networking; help people to meet likeminded people; create supportive environments in which to meet people with similar support needs that ultimately could lead to change in social attitudes; and help older people to become more accepted and involved in local communities. The project was evaluated via feedback from volunteers and service users through an iterative process that meant that both groups were involved in the future planning of the project as well as its implementation and evaluation.

The main issues the project addressed in terms of social isolation were that: it gave socially isolated older people an opportunity to talk to someone, to have a sounding board, and to look forward to a visit every week; it provided a link with the outside world, which was particularly important for older people who were largely house bound; people started to engage socially outside of the organised activities, people visited each other and arranged outings independently of the project; and that participants gained confidence, with project staff noticing that people were better able to carry out daily tasks such as going to pick up a paper, and were more willing to try new things. The project also provided an opportunity for general health-improvement initiatives like falls prevention, increasing physical activity and increasing uptake of flu vaccinations to be promoted with older age participants.

The success of the project appeared to be rooted in the fact that it sought to reduce social isolation in a vulnerable group through addressing not only their individual needs for social contact, but also by looking at how this could be expanded to the wider community and by overcoming some of the structural barriers:

- Transport, and in particular transport for those with a disability, was provided.
- Social groups provided the social activity people wanted, for example a men's group offered a hot meal in a pub.
- Support was offered in people's homes when needed.
- Support in terms of befriending gave people confidence and helped them to overcome some of the anxiety that had developed with living alone.

The project took many of its referrals from mental health services, so many clients were already experiencing depression, and feedback from both volunteers and service users indicated that in these, and other participants, it helped alleviate the stress, anxiety and depression that often accompanies isolation.

Participation in meaningful activity

'A meaningful role can provide a sense of purpose and identity, a reason to get out of bed in the morning and something to care about' (Age Concern and the Mental Health Foundation 2006: 30). For some older age adults, identity can be lost at the point at which employment or family demands diminish. Only half of all retired people say they wanted to stop working, and over a third say they felt forced to stop (Department for Work and Pensions 2005). Older people comment that being forced to retire against one's will has a very negative effect on their mental health and well-being (Age Concern and the Mental Health Foundation 2006).

The consequences of not having meaningful participation in later life are varied and can mean that older people's abilities and skills are not valued or appreciated, their skills are often under-utilised, and there is a reduction in physical and mental activities leading in some cases to a decline in abilities, discrimination and poor community cohesion.

A number of initiatives have sought to address the problems produced by lack of meaningful participation:

- The *Sure Start to Later Life* is a national initiative aiming to provide a single access point to a range of services older people may need, for example housing or social benefits, but will also include opportunities for volunteering, lifelong learning and social activities (Social Exclusion Unit 2006).
- Pre-retirement courses and support can be offered in the workplace or in community settings and involve planning for having time, signposting to activities, as well as practical advice about pensions. The workplace is also a key setting to address the whole issue of work-life balance so that people do not find themselves at 50+ having dedicated a lifetime to work with little other interest or ambition.
- Consultation forums, and civic and political duties have assumed greater importance in recent years. Local authority areas forums, either real or virtual, where older citizens are invited to shape service provision are now commonplace. Indeed, Councils use the engagement of older people as part of their performance assessment, giving the opportunity for greater civic involvement (Hatton-Yeo 2006). Civic involvement is in turn seen as a key measure of social capital.

Case study 2: older people's experiences of volunteering

This case study draws on the findings from two projects conducted across the north-east that sought to draw on the experiences of older people who had been involved in volunteering in a range of settings and offering a range of services. One was a collaborative project between the University of Newcastle-upon-Tyne and Age Concern Newcastle (Baines, Lie and Wheelock 2006), and the other was a project looking at examples of older male volunteering across the north-east (Cutts 2006). The lessons learned from these projects highlight what motivates older people to volunteer, the challenges they face and the perceived health benefits of volunteering.

In each of these two projects the type of volunteering activity undertaken was varied and included befriending and visiting, providing transport to others to attend appointments or social events, cooking and serving food in a range of settings, providing administrative support to organisations, fund raising and management tasks, as well as representing older people on consultative groups. This was carried out within a variety of settings and a range of organisations. In addition to the formal volunteering evaluated in these two projects, volunteers played other roles within their communities and families that were described as informal volunteering, for example looking after grandchildren, shopping for neighbours or being active in community task groups.

The project found that while there are some common motivators for volunteers across age groups, there are some issues that are particularly pertinent to older volunteers, and that whilst younger volunteers are keen to gain experience, older volunteers are keen to pass on the experience they already have. Younger volunteers also see it as an opportunity to add to a curriculum vitae, whereas for older volunteers gaining access to paid employment is less important. In summary, the motivation for older people volunteering included:

- Being a useful member of society.
- Putting something back into the community.
- Meeting new people.
- Personal learning growth.
- To fill a void left by retirement.
- Something to fill their time.

The challenges they faced were: lack of access to transport, especially for those with mobility problems; safety issues and fear of crime; age discrimination, with insurance companies imposing age restrictions on volunteers' activities; lack of training, as they were sometimes viewed by some organisations as too frail or not worth investing in; the professionalising of volunteering and the rise of a contract culture as organisations seek to meet the emerging governance requirements.

Some of the issues identified in these projects are common across all health-improvement interventions with older people, for example access to transport and fear of crime; however, there are some that are particularly pertinent to volunteering. An increasing emphasis on governance has made the professionalisation of volunteers almost inevitable. Statutory and voluntary sector organisations are increasingly developing volunteer policies and contracts which include occupational health checks, Criminal Records Bureau checks and requirements to undergo extensive training and induction programmes. The governance structures can be seen as prohibitive to older, and in particular older and disabled, people. The project highlighted that older volunteers described increased life satisfaction, forgetting their own troubles whilst helping others. They also experienced:

- A feeling of satisfaction at doing something that might make a difference.
- Increased self confidence.
- A sense of autonomy.
- Keeping active and learning new tasks.

It is also clear from these projects that volunteering doesn't just help improve the mental health of individuals, but also adds value to their local communities.

Improving physical health

The relationship between physical and mental health is complex, but it is well established that poor physical health and poor mental health are linked (National Institute for

Mental Health England 2005). When we have better mental health our physical health outcomes and recovery rates improve, and when our physical health is good we are less prone to common mental health problems such as anxiety and depression. Physical activity has an important role to play in the development and maintenance of both good physical and good mental health, and is increasingly promoted as a vehicle for improving both in older age. The evidence base for the benefits of physical activity in all stages of life is expanding, but shows that increasing physical activity in people of any age group, but especially older people, can improve quality of life, improve both physical and mental health, and reduce the risk of falls.

The promotion of independence and a healthy active life amongst older people has been the cornerstone of a number of key policy documents, including the *National Service Framework for Older People* (Department of Health 2001b) and *Better Government for Older People Programme* (Cabinet Office 2001). The *National Service Framework for Older People* states that ' ... any form of social, physical or mental activity is good for health and well-being. The adoption of a more physically active lifestyle can add years to life for previously inactive older people, but perhaps more importantly, physical activity can significantly enhance mobility and independence and improve quality of life' (Department of Health 2001b: 110).

Case study 3: active ageing

The Newcastle Active Ageing Programme was developed to promote physical activity and well-being amongst older people in the neighbourhood renewal areas of Newcastle-upon-Tyne. The Active Ageing Programme brought together a range of people with expertise in developing services for older people. This included people from both the statutory and voluntary sectors, along with people from the community of older people in Newcastle-upon-Tyne.

The Active Ageing Programme specifically sought to:

- Increase capacity in disadvantaged communities and in so doing contribute to building confidence and social cohesion.
- Reduce social isolation and promote physical and mental well-being amongst targeted groups.
- Promote independence amongst older people.
- Increase opportunities for older people to demonstrate that they are not a burden.
- Recognise that older people are part of the solution.
- Enhance networks and links between strategies and services for older people by making better use of resources.
- Include older people in local policy-making and in decisions about local service provision.

The scheme sought to achieve these outcomes through provision of a range of innovative and challenging activities and programmes of work to support older people. These activities ranged from provision of taster sessions in a diverse range of activities provided at local venues, including tai chi and bowls, to challenging, one-off outdoor activities such as abseiling, as well as gardening groups, the development of a website featuring local walks, and a range of instructor courses.

Evaluation of the Programme identified a range of factors associated with success in engaging people in physical activities as well as lessons for the future (Crosland *et al*. 2005).

Successes of the Programme:

- The opportunities to meet new people and mix with others were the main reasons older people participated in the Programme.
- Trying out new skills had an important impact in improving self-confidence amongst participants.
- Efforts to build capacity for delivery of exercise programmes for older people led to 30 new instructors being trained in the first two years of the Programme. This included walk leaders, fitness instructors and chair-based exercise instructors, many of whom were themselves retired.
- A number of older participants in the programme went on to become involved in planning and steering specific activities.
- Lessons from the Programme were fed back and disseminated to a wider audience through a series of one-off events and presentations.
- Active Ageing provided added value and helped build social capital through the development of a strong programme team and steering group. This strong network developed over time.
- Participants' quality of life was enhanced through promoting companionship through group activities, providing new goals and challenges to promote a sense of purpose, through celebration of success and achievement, and through promoting a sense of self-worth by encouraging older people to express themselves and give voice to their views and experiences.
- Positioning the Active Ageing Programme outside any one organisation allowed the steering group to try out new ideas free from conventional sources of resistance.
- Trust and openness amongst the steering group helped promote a climate that allowed members to reflect on relative success and limitations and maximised learning from the Programme.
- The Programme successfully demonstrated the abilities of older people and in so doing challenged popular misconceptions about older people and ageing.

Lessons learned

Lessons centred on the need to target and cater for the most disadvantaged members of society as many of those who were recruited in the early days were those who were already part of social networks rather than the hard to reach groups sought. There was resistance from some staff in sheltered housing, leisure services and education which had to be addressed and which led to recommendations about the need for education and training of a diverse range of staff to overcome barriers in the future. Perhaps the main lessons, though, were that much can be achieved through the involvement of older people in all stages of development, implementation and steering the project, and that this approach is most successful when older people from diverse backgrounds and with a wide range of experiences are involved. Indeed, an inclusive approach that draws in people with different physical and mental health needs offers the best opportunity for normalisation of services, reducing discrimination and protecting older people from a range of mental health problems in later life.

Addressing discrimination

Discrimination is the experience of many people in many different settings. Age discrimination has a negative impact on mental health in later life by making people feel undervalued, not respected and misunderstood. Both direct and indirect discrimination are experienced by people as they get older. Age discrimination is the most common form of prejudice experienced in later life (Age Concern and the Mental Health Foundation 2006). Age can be a barrier to access to services, including mental health services which have separate structures for people of working age, i.e. those under 65, compared to those of older people. Older people may also have restricted access to benefits on the basis of their age.

Whilst age discrimination may be the most common form of discrimination experienced by older people, some experience additional discrimination including that based on gender and ethnicity.

Case study 4: a cardiac rehabilitation programme

Westgate Heartbeat was a project set up in the West End of Newcastle to work with black and minority ethnic (BME) groups within the Westgate New Deals for Communities area (Crosland *et al.* 2004). The aim of the project was to improve access to information about primary prevention of heart disease and to provide culturally sensitive cardiac rehabilitation programmes. There were no age parameters put on access to the project; however, almost all participants were aged over 55. There was no express aim to improve mental health amongst this group but, as we shall see later, this was one of the consequences of certain aspects of the programme from which we can learn lessons about how to reduce discrimination in marginalised groups.

The project team consisted of a cardiac rehabilitation nurse, several community development workers from within the BME community, trainee development workers and a team secretary.

The project took a long time to get up and running as it proved difficult to recruit bilingual workers from within the community as many of the younger people from within the BME community had not learned the first language of their parents and grandparents. Added to this, a lack of confidence in many older people in the community in speaking and communicating in English largely excluded many older people from applying. Once recruited, it then took time for the development workers to be trained. When up and running it soon became clear that existing cardiac rehabilitation services were insensitive to the needs of members of the BME community. Of particular note was the timing of sessions that clashed with the religious needs of participants, mixed gender groups were unacceptable to many, assumptions made by professionals about lifestyles, diet and knowledge of anatomy and physiology were often seen as insulting, and the use of interpreters in sessions proved to be cumbersome.

All of these factors, plus a fear of racial abuse and crime, provided a barrier to participants accessing mainstream services. A number of efforts were then made to locate more culturally sensitive services within local communities, with mixed success. One notable success here was a women's dance group led by a South African nurse. All of the women were over the age of 55, only a few were confident speaking English, all had previously been difficult to engage and all were socially isolated. Most had either pre-existing coronary heart disease or were identified as at high risk of a future cardiac event.

The group met weekly at a local women's centre and all attended regularly to meet socially, undertake an exercise programme and build confidence. Whilst the exercise programme was similar to others used for cardiac rehabilitation, describing this as a dance session had more meaning for the women involved. There were no requirements to dress in any particular way and once set up the group was closed to new participants at their request.

The session was evaluated with the support of interpreters and the women reported that as the weeks went by, their confidence, knowledge and awareness of a range of health issues had increased, they felt more part of a local community and the lessons they learned were being passed on to other women and girls within their community (Visram *et al.* 2007).

Participants were keen to continue with the group beyond the life of the project and actively sought alternative avenues of support for this. The power of the group lay in the shared experiences and opportunities for mutual support. Many of the women felt empowered by their experiences and reported much more positive attitudes to their health. The lessons learned from the group were fed back into the development of cardiac and other rehabilitation services and recommendations for training and development of staff were made.

Reducing poverty

Financial security is critical to mental health and well-being in later life as it ensures that older people have access to the goods and resources necessary to maintain good health, for example essentials such as adequate housing, food and warmth, and the non-essentials that improve quality of life such as social activities, newspapers, magazines and the occasional treat. However, poverty is a fact of life for many older people with two-thirds of pensioners relying on their state pension and benefits for at least half of their income (Department for Work and Pensions 2005). This is much higher for pensioners living in disadvantaged areas. Women, carers and people from minority ethnic communities are particularly disadvantaged by the pension system in the UK (Adams, Carter and Schäfer 2006). Poverty earlier on in life can also lead to increased likelihood of poverty in later life. Poverty can exacerbate existing health problems and create new ones.

A lack of access to the resources that many of us take for granted can have long-term psychological effects on people, increasing stress and anxiety whilst at the same time reducing self-esteem and resilience making them more vulnerable to depression following bereavement or other significant life events. Poverty compounds existing inequalities and can lead to social exclusion. It is estimated that 20 percent of older people are excluded from developing social relationships and participating in cultural and civic activities because of poverty (Age Concern and the Mental Health Foundation 2006).

Access to financial resources is important in minimising stress and improving quality of life for older people. The changes required to take all older people out of poverty would require substantial political will and intervention that is beyond the scope of the discussion presented here. However, there are efforts that can be made at a local level to ameliorate the situation for the poorest older people. Up to 40 percent of those entitled to pension credit fail to claim it each year, amounting to £2.1 billion in unclaimed benefits. A similar percentage fails to claim council tax benefits. Supporting older people to claim the benefits to which they are entitled can have a big impact not only on the lives of individuals but also on the communities within which they live. Moffat and Scambler (2008), in a small-scale primary care-based study that offered welfare rights advice to men and women over the age of 60, found that the additional money obtained by individual claimants increased the affordability of necessities, helped people cope with emergencies and reduced levels of stress and anxiety.

Case study 5: an information and advice service

In 2000, with the help of a grant from the Northern Rock Foundation, Age Concern in Gateshead set up an information and advice service for older people across the borough of Gateshead, which has nine out of 22 wards that fall within the top 10 percent of the most deprived wards in England. Gateshead also has a higher than national average number of residents over the age of 60 years. The services available through this scheme were delivered in a range of settings and incorporated a number of different initiatives, all of which had the primary aim of supporting older people in accessing benefits to which they were entitled.

Services offered included:

- Telephone advice during normal working hours.
- E-mail service and drop-in sessions.
- A home visiting service for housebound clients or clients who may have caring responsibilities.
- A hospital advice service.
- Weekly advice sessions in a local rehabilitation unit.
- An annual benefits take-up campaign called Your Rights Week in conjunction with Age Concern England.
- Regular tax surgeries in conjunction with Tax for Older People.
- Promotional talks and events to groups and the public at large in places from the Metrocentre and Asda to community centres and bowling clubs.
- Visits to sheltered housing to give benefits talks every Monday afternoon, covering the whole borough in a year, in conjunction with the local authority and Department for Work and Pensions.
- Provision of a rolling programme of advice sessions in libraries across the borough.

In addition, the information and advice service entered into a partnership with Tyne & Wear Black Housing Project (TWBHP) to try and encourage contact from BME elders and, as a trial, set up four joint sessions based at Millennium House in Gateshead. TWBHP provided translation services and widened its remit to include advice for the under 50s for these sessions, as the service was unable to afford translation any other way.

Over a four-year period between 2001 and 2005 a total of £3,050,870 of new grants and benefits was obtained on behalf of all older people living in Gateshead. Some of this had remained unclaimed for years. This made a huge difference to the people concerned at an individual level – and also meant that a further £3 million was brought into the local economy to be spent on local goods and services. In mental health terms it opened up opportunities for recipients who could now afford to pay for transport and thus access a wider range of services and social networks. Not only did it assist those who were already facing mental health difficulties, but it also helped protect against further such problems in the future.

Discussion

Mental health promotion for older people requires a complex set of activities that focus not only on the needs of the individual but also on the needs of the communities within which they live and the structural barriers they face in their everyday lives. Mental health promotion works best when it tackles issues at all of these levels. As the examples presented here demonstrate, any one set of activities can address a number of issues identified as important to the improvement of mental health in later life (Age Concern and the Mental Health Foundation 2006). So, whilst the Active Ageing Programme was focused primarily on the improvement of the physical health of participants, it also offered an opportunity for developing social relationships between some of the more isolated participants and meaningful participation for others, through their involvement in the steering group or as physical activity advisers. Furthermore, it fostered the development of stronger communities within which older people live and at the same time it sought to uncover and address structural barriers such as the negative attitudes of those working with older people in sheltered accommodation. In a similar vein, Westgate Heartbeat, which at first glance appeared to be a focused project looking at cardiac rehabilitation in the BME community in a disadvantaged part of Newcastle-upon-Tyne, actually identified multiple sources of direct and indirect discrimination and at the same time helped strengthen social networks and support structures within these marginalised communities. Without these efforts to build support and address structural barriers older people face in improving their mental health and well-being, efforts to improve mental health at an individual level may well be set up to fail and in so doing could have the opposite effect to that sought.

There is much to be learned from the approaches adopted by many of the third sector organisations that developed and led four of the examples given here. The adoption of an holistic approach to health improvement such as that deployed in the Active Ageing Programme, which sought to improve physical activity levels in older people whilst at the same time facilitating social contacts and improving participants' self confidence, embeds mental health promotion as a central part of all health improvement activities and not as something to be addressed separately. This approach appears to be even more successful when it adds value to the local community, e.g. the Gateshead Welfare Advice Service helped boost the local economy and therefore ensured that local services were maintained. The Good Companions Project increased the number of local volunteers within the community, which had the added benefit of more active older people to engage in meaningful activities within their communities.

Addressing the needs of communities rather than just individuals, however, requires working across agencies and across disciplines in health and social care and into other groups and stakeholders, e.g. welfare rights workers, leisure services staff and others in both the statutory and voluntary sectors. This brings with it further challenges. The partnership ideal has underpinned public policies for over a decade; however, true partnership working requires a great deal of effort on the part of practitioners and managers in addition to support from the highest level within organisations. For mental health improvement the time-limited project-based approach, i.e. short-term funding that is common in health promotion, means that this is often the easiest area to cut in hard times or when policy changes are brought in. This is true of all prevention and health promotion initiatives which tend to be dictated by current policy imperatives that disappear when political champions move on. Ensuring longer-term and more mainstream funding may be essential for health promotion initiatives as this allows sufficient time for the measurement of success, or otherwise. The paradox here is that mainstream funding is often dictated by policy and predicated on the belief that an intervention works and therefore on-going evaluation is rarely built in. Once in place it is then difficult to retract the money. Recent examples include the introduction of health trainers (Department of Health 2004), who have now been mainstreamed in many organisations but whose effectiveness has not been robustly tested, and whilst there is no evidence to say that they are effective, nor is there evidence to say that they are not. An additional benefit to mainstream funding is that staff are more likely to stay in the system, thus building capacity for mental health improvement. Any changes to funding arrangements, however, need to recognise that there are risks, i.e. mainstreaming can stifle innovation as people are less likely to take risks and it can marginalise those organisations that often do it best such as those in the third sector. There are lessons here for more recent policy initiatives such as the *National Dementia Strategy* in England (Department of Health 2009), which places more emphasis on staying well but does not really indicate how this can be sustained in the long term and how its impact will be assessed.

Evaluation of mental health promotion initiatives

The complex nature of mental health promotion presents a number of challenges for evaluating what works and for whom. In particular, without a clear definition of mental health and clear models for understanding mental health promotion, evaluation is almost impossible. This is particularly important given the current move towards more partnership and collaborative working, where partners may have different ideas and understanding of the issues and may have different aims for evaluation of interventions. Evaluations of any initiatives for older people can be made even more difficult by the fact that many older people may not identify themselves as such and thus may not participate either in the intervention itself or in its evaluation. Collectively, these issues often mean that mental health promotion initiatives need clear inclusion and exclusion criteria as well as clarity of aims and a realistic assessment of what can be achieved.

Traditional approaches to evaluation have tended to be either very simplistic and focused on the collection of routine data about throughput or have used more complex experimental methods focused on outcomes. Such approaches provide a decontextualised account of who uses the services or what effect it has when measured against a narrowly defined measureable outcome or outcomes. They do not indicate how or what elements of a complex intervention works and in what circumstances, or if it is acceptable to older people within the context of their everyday lives, which are often the questions that are important to both older people and those who commission services (Smith *et al.* 2009).

A range of evaluation models that capture the dynamic and complex nature of health improvement initiatives is required. Action-oriented approaches that can evaluate change as it happens and from the perspectives of different stakeholders were used to evaluate the case study projects presented in this chapter. Whilst historically these approaches have not been common in health promotion settings (Whitehead, Taket and Smith 2003), they were valuable here not least because they captured change as it happened. The additional value of these action-oriented approaches is that they commonly work with participants as equal partners in the research or evaluation process (Hart and Bond 1995), and in the cases presented in the chapter allowed the voices of older people to be heard. Other approaches can also add value to the evaluation of mental health promotion initiatives. This includes case study methods that allow for in-depth exploration of the case (here the case being either a project or community) under investigation and therefore 'fit' with health promotion principles that seek to improve health at the individual, community and structural levels (Yin 2003). Pawson and Tilley's (1997) context, process, mechanism approach is also useful as it can capture the individual elements of an intervention that appear to make a difference even if the intervention as a whole fails to demonstrate quantifiable change. All of these approaches allow for the use of a range of methods for data capture that not only look at the process and effects of an intervention but also centralise the experiences of older people.

Education and training for mental health promotion

The examples outlined in this chapter demonstrate that interventions to improve mental health in later life are complex and involve a wide range of partners. They also illustrate how staff working in a range of public, private and third sector organisations need to understand mental health promotion. For example, for the Active Ageing Programme to have maximum impact, staff in health services, care homes and leisure centres would have benefited from a better understanding of how to promote positive mental health, and older people themselves would have benefited from better understanding and support for participation in decision-making about the project. However, training in mental health promotion is not widely available and mental health promotion is rarely a feature of public health education programmes in universities and colleges (North East Teaching Public Health Network 2008).

Education and training is needed for a wide range of individuals and groups working in different parts and at different levels of the health and social care system as well as for those working across organisations. This includes managers, commissioners, care staff, health promotion staff, policy-makers, educators and older people themselves. Specific training needs include:

- Those working in generalist services such as primary care staff or those working in nursing and care homes who regularly come into contact with older people. Their training needs would centre on developing an understanding of the needs of older people and of models for promoting mental health.
- Service commissioners who need to understand how to measure the effectiveness of complex interventions so that they can commission the best services for their local populations, i.e. services that support positive mental health in later life.
- Older community members to ensure that they feel confident and empowered to influence others in their decision-making about service development.
- Mental health promotion specialists who need to develop leadership skills to ensure that the best mental health promotion policies and practices are implemented for the benefit of local older people and that other staff have the skills and capacity to support this.
- People who make local policies and plan services such as town planners and leisure service leaders who need to understand how their work impacts upon the mental health and well-being of older people.
- Academic public health staff who need the theoretical knowledge and skills relating to mental health promotion so that they can support the development of others in adapting these to their own practice.

Conclusion

As the number of older people increases in the UK and across the world and more effort is directed towards prevention rather than cure, mental health promotion in later life will become a more pressing issue for all workers dealing with the needs of older people. However, mental health promotion has not been seen as a priority for those providing services for older people, and examples of interventions to promote mental health in this age group are uncommon. Furthermore, mental health promotion for older people is not seen as a priority for those working with health improvement settings.

As this chapter has demonstrated, most of the successful efforts to address mental health promotion in later life carried out in the north-east of England have been those developed and led by third sector organisations such as Age Concern. The dearth of literature on this topic suggests that a similar picture would be found across the UK. This lack of evidence mirrors the lack of services to support mental health promotion programmes for this age group. The range of mental health problems people face in later life, many of which are covered in this book, point to a need for a wide range of services that are flexible enough to accommodate the complex range of mental health and mental health promotion needs that older people experience. Holistic models for health improvement are also required to integrate mental health improvement into all health promotion services and improvement interventions, so that mental health improvement becomes a central feature of health improvement in later life rather than the add-on that it is currently. Perhaps most importantly, though the examples here illustrate that it does not matter at what stage of life an individual is, positive mental health is important and health improvement can be achieved, and this is best approached through the involvement of older people at all stages of planning and implementation of interventions to promote positive mental health.

References

Adams, L., Carter, K. and Schäfer, L. (2006) *Equal pay review survey 2005 Working Paper Series No42*, London: Equal Opportunities Commission.

Age Concern and the Mental Health Foundation (2006) *Promoting mental health and well-being in later-life: A first report of the UK inquiry into mental health and well-being in later life*, London: Age Concern and the Mental Health Foundation. Available: www.mhilli.org (accessed 4 February 2010).

——(2008) *Literature review on mental health promotion in later life. Completed for the UK Inquiry into mental health and well-being in later life*, London: Age Concern and the Mental Health Foundation.

Age Concern Gateshead (2004) *Good Companions evaluation report*, Gateshead: Age Concern Gateshead.

Alexander, T. (2002) *A bright future for all, promoting mental health in education*, London: The Mental Health Foundation.

Baines, S., Lie, M. and Wheelock, J. (2006) *Volunteering, Self Help and Citizenship in later life – A collaborative project by Age Concern Newcastle and The University of Newcastle-upon-Tyne*, Newcastle: Age Concern.

Cabinet Office (2001) *Better Government for Older People Programme*, London: HMSO.

Cole, M.G. and Dendukuri, N. (2004) 'The feasibility and effectiveness of brief interventions to prevent depression in older subjects: a systematic review', *International Journal of Geriatric Psychiatry*, 19: 1019–25.

Cooper, H., Arber, S., Fee, L. and Ginn, J. (1999) *Making it happen – A guide to delivering Mental Health Promotion*, London, Department of Health.

Crosland, A., Unsworth, J., Prudhoe, A. and Mode, A. (2005) *Evaluation of the Active Ageing Scheme*, Newcastle-upon-Tyne: Northumbria University.

Crosland, A., Unsworth, J., Visram, S., Mode, A. and Harrington, B. (2004) *Evaluation of Westgate Heartbeat*, Newcastle-upon-Tyne: Northumbria University.

Cutts, A. (2006) *Older male volunteers in social care and community action*, Volunteering in the Third Age (VITA).

Department of Health (2001a) *Making it happen – A guide to delivering Mental Health Promotion*, London: Department of Health.

——(2001b) *National Service Framework for Older People*, London: Department of Health.

——(2004) *Choosing health: making healthy choices easier*, London: Department of Health.

——(2009) *Living well with dementia, a National Dementia Strategy*, London: Department of Health.

Department for Work and Pensions (2005) *Opportunity age: meeting the challenges of ageing in the 21st Century Volumes 1 & 2*, London: Department for Work and Pensions.

Freidli, L., Oliver, C., Tidyman, M. and Ward, G. (2007) *Mental Health Improvement: evidence based messages to promote mental well-being*, NHS Scotland.

Hart, E. and Bond, M. (1995) *Action research for Health and Social Care*, Maidenhead: Open University Press.

Hatton-Yeo, A. (2006) *Intergenerational programmes: An introduction and examples of practice*, The Beth Johnson Foundation.

Lomas, J. (1998) 'Social capital and health – implications for public health and epidemiology', *Social Science and Medicine* 47 (9): 1181–88.

McDonald, G. and O'Hara, K. (1998) *Ten elements of mental health promotion and demotion: implications for practice*, Society of Health Education and Promotion Specialists.

McNicholas, J., Gilbey, A., Rennie, A. and Dono, J. (2005) 'Pet ownership and human health: A brief overview of evidence and issue', *British Medical Journal*, 331: 1252–55.

Moffat, S. and Scambler, G. (2008) 'Can welfare-rights advice targeted at older people reduce social exclusion?' *Ageing and Society*, 28: 875–99.

National Institute for Mental Health England (2005) *Making it possible: improving mental health and well-being in England*, London: National Institute for Mental Health England.

North East Teaching Public Health Network (2008) *Phase two Mapping of Public Health Education*. Available: www.TPHN.org.uk (accessed 4 February 2010).

Nurse, J. (2009) *Creating Flourishing Communities: a public mental health framework for building resilience, reducing inequalities and developing well-being*, London: Department of Health.

Pawson, R. and Tilley, N. (1997) *Realistic Evaluation*, London: Sage.

Social Exclusion Unit (2006) *A Sure Start to later life: Ending inequalities for older people*, London: Office of the Deputy Prime Minister.

Smith, K., Crosland, A., Wallace, A. and Haining, S. (2009) *Commissioning for public health*, UK Public Health Association 17th Annual Conference, Brighton.

Visram, S., Crosland, A., Unsworth, J. and Long, S. (2007) 'Engaging women from South Asian communities in cardiac rehabilitation', *British Journal of Community Nursing*, 12 (1): 13–18.

Whitehead, D., Taket, A. and Smith, P. (2003) 'Action research in health promotion', *Health Education Journal*, 62 (1): 2–22.

World Health Organization (1986) *Ottawa Charter for health promotion*, Ottawa: WHO.

——(2005) *Mental health declaration and action plan for Europe: Facing the challenges, building solutions*, Helsinki: WHO Europe.

——(2007) *Mental Health: strengthening mental health promotion*, Fact sheet No. 220. Available: www.who.int/mediacentre/factsheets/fs220/en/ (accessed 9 April 2010).

Yin, R. (2003) *Case Study research: design and methods*, Thousand Oaks, CA: Sage.

Part 2

Clinical contexts

4 Anxiety and depression in older people

Georgina Charlesworth and Janet Carter

Key messages

- Mixed anxiety and depression is a common presentation to older people's community mental health teams (CMHTs), more prevalent than either 'pure' anxiety or depression, but has not yet received the attention of policy-makers.
- Somatic complaints are a common presenting symptom for anxiety meaning diagnosis is frequently missed.
- Antidepressants with anxiolytic properties have a useful role but under-treatment of depression and anxiety in primary care is common.
- Older people's CMHTs often need to work in partnership with other health or social care providers to adequately intervene with older people with clinically significant anxiety and depression.
- Family and social (including religious) networks, health, and attitudes to ageing and mental health need to be taken into account when care planning.

Introduction

Definitions

Depression is characterised by low mood and loss of interest in life. The symptoms of depressive disorders are pervasive, and can impact on all areas of a person's day-to-day living. Biological symptoms include loss of appetite and changes to sleep patterns. Psychological symptoms include feelings of guilt and a sense of hopelessness while behavioural symptoms include withdrawal from others and reduced engagement with activities of daily living.

The characteristics of anxiety in later life include anxious mood, tension and non-specific somatic complaints such as dizziness, shakiness and nausea. Autonomic hyper-arousal is common and often accompanied by anxious ruminations over health or 'free-floating' worries in relation to trivial matters which are often recognised as irrational. The extent to which anxiety in older and younger people is qualitatively different has been an area of debate, and has yet to be resolved (Bryant et al. 2008).

Demographics and prevalence

The rate of depression in older people has been surveyed in nine sites across Europe by the EURODEP consortium (Copeland et al. 2004). In a meta-analysis of GMS-AGECAT data from 13,808 participants aged 65 or above, the rate of depression was 12 percent. There were both geographical variations and a gender bias. For example, the rate for depression was 17.3 percent in London compared with 10 percent in Liverpool, and was 14 percent for women compared with 8.6 percent for men. For residents of care homes the prevalence of depression can be as much as 40 percent (Age Concern and the Mental Health Foundation 2007).

From a review of prevalence studies of anxiety in older people, Bryant and colleagues (Bryant *et al.* 2008) suggested that the prevalence rates for anxiety range from 1.2 percent to 14 percent in community samples and 1 percent to 28 percent in clinical settings. The wide range of estimates may be due to methodological variations, such as differences in the 'status' of anxiety within diagnostic classification systems where forms of anxiety are subsumed under depression and not 'counted' if depression is present. Other methodological differences include the threshold at which anxiety symptoms reach clinical significance and methods for distinguishing between somatic symptoms and psychological distress. The overall rate of anxiety disorders rises dramatically for particular groups, for example 23.5 percent in carers of people with dementia (Mahoney *et al.* 2005) and 28 percent of admissions to a stroke unit (Astrom 1996). Rates are also high for the housebound, those resident in nursing care and people with chronic medical conditions.

Where Generalized Anxiety Disorder (GAD) has been included in studies of anxiety, it has generally been found more prevalent than phobic disorders and panic. Obsessive Compulsive Disorders and Post-Traumatic Stress Disorder are considered rare (see Bryant *et al.* 2008 for a review). Flint (2005) suggested that pure GAD in older people is evenly split between those with chronic problems commencing early in life and those with onset for the first time in late life. The most consistent finding regarding late-life GAD, however, is its high level of co-morbidity with depression.

The co-existence of clinically significant symptoms of both anxiety and depression frequently prompts a diagnosis of a mixed anxiety depressive state. A recent longitudinal Dutch community-based study in an older population (58–85 years at baseline) demonstrated clinically relevant anxiety in 10.8 percent, 5.4 percent with anxiety and 6 percent with a mixed picture (Vink *et al.* 2009). Authors of the MRC Cognitive Function and Ageing Study (CFAS; Kvaal *et al.* 2008) suggested that 'pure' disorders of anxiety and depression are relatively rare in comparison with the combined state of anxiety and depression. Using the GMS-AGECAT system, Kvaal and colleagues found that the overall prevalence of overlapping anxiety or depressive disorders was 8.4 percent. As for depression, the prevalence was higher in women than men and with a strong association with disability.

Synthesis of key literature

If anxiety and depression overlap to such a great extent, what is the relationship between them, and what are the implications for treatment? In terms of risk factors, there are more similarities than differences between anxiety and depression (Vink *et al.* 2008). The overlap of symptomatology has also led some to suggest that GAD and depression are merely different aspects of the same illness.

In terms of treatments, the high rate of co-morbidity of depression and anxiety supports the use of medications with both anxiolytic and antidepressant effects. The evidence base is limited but where depressive symptoms predominate or where anxiety is secondary to depression then antidepressants are probably the main treatment of choice.

Studies of these in older adults are limited but Selective Serotonin Reuptake Inhibitors (SSRIs) such as Citalopram and Venlafaxine are effective and well tolerated (Baldwin *et al.* 2005). In a review of 18 studies of the efficacy of antidepressants in older people, Mukai and Tampi (2009) suggest that the dual-action agents (tri-cyclic antidepressants and serotonin-noradrenaline reuptake inhibitors) do not appear to confer any additional benefits in efficacy over SSRIs. Other treatments may include the short-term judicious use of Benzodiazepines which are effective for anxiety symptoms but increase the risk of falls, sedation, tolerance and dependence.

More recent pharmacological approaches include the introduction of more specific treatments for GAD including Buspirone and Pregabalin. A large randomized controlled trial supports the tolerability and efficacy of the latter for use in GAD (Montgomery *et al.* 2008).

In terms of psychological interventions, depression has again received greater attention than either anxiety or mixed states. Findings for depression suggest that psychological therapies are as efficacious in older people as they are in younger cohorts, and that there is no clear benefit of any one psychotherapeutic approach (Scogin *et al.* 2005). For anxiety, the limited evidence base points towards cognitive behavioural therapy (CBT) and relaxation training (Ayers *et al.* 2007).

Policy considerations

Whereas epidemiological research and clinical experience point towards the importance of considering mixed depression and anxiety states, policy guidance focuses on either depression alone, or depression and anxiety separately.

The *National Service Framework for Older People* (Department of Health 2001) included depression as one of its targets within standard 7, 'Mental Health of Older People', whereas anxiety was notable by its absence. Indeed, throughout the *National Service Framework for Older People*, the term 'anxiety' is used only once (Department of Health 2001: 73, para. 7.17).

The *National Service Framework for Older People* outlines the treatment of depression as follows:

- Making the diagnosis and giving the person an explanation of their symptoms.
- Assessment of risk, especially suicidal intent, and looking for co-existing physical problems, especially possible dementia or physical illness.
- Giving information about the likely prognosis and options for packages of care.
- Making appropriate referrals to help with the fears and worries, distress, practical and financial issues that will affect the person and their carer.
- Prescribing antidepressant medicines.
- Offering psychological therapies alongside antidepressant drug treatment.

(Department of Health 2001: 95, para. 7.27)

The *National Service Framework for Older People* emphasises the importance of specialist mental health services, and recommends referral to such services (Department of Health 2001: 95, para. 7.30) for those with suspected depression where:

- Diagnosis is uncertain.
- There are complex symptoms, for example multiple physical problems.

- There is a suicide risk. Risk factors include past attempt, painful medical condition, bereavement, severity of current depression, alcohol dependence, being male and, for some, transition from employment.
- There has been an inadequate response to first line treatments.
- The older person has psychotic symptoms such as delusions.

Since the *National Service Framework for Older People* (Department of Health 2001), the National Institute for Health and Clinical Excellence (NICE) has produced guidance for depression (National Collaborating Centre for Mental Health 2007) and for anxiety (National Collaborating Centre for Primary Care 2007). Both these guidelines are intended for all adults over the age of 18, and in the depression guidance a clear distinction is drawn between those over and under 65 years of age for both pharmacological and psychosocial interventions. The anxiety guidance acknowledges the challenge to establishing efficacy for older people as many trials limit the inclusion of over 65s.

Overall, policy guidance supports the use of similar treatment strategies for older people as are available for younger adults. However, these recommendations are made without reference to the common significant events and circumstances for older populations such as bereavement, physical health difficulties and providing family care to ailing spouses. NICE has recently produced guidelines for the treatment of depression in the context of chronic physical health difficulties (www.nice.org.uk/cg91). In contrast to the earlier guidance, guideline 91 acknowledges the co-occurrence of depression and anxiety. The recommendations made are that depression should be the focus of treatment when depression is accompanied by symptoms of anxiety, but that anxiety disorders should be the primary focus for treatment when co-morbid with either depression or depressive symptoms.

Applying principles

About the team

The cases discussed in this chapter were seen in mental health services for people aged 65 and above in an outer London borough. The borough has a population of nearly a quarter of a million people and, at 17.5 percent, the proportion of residents who are over 65 is higher than in any other London borough. The area has, within living memory, shifted from being administered by a rural county council to being part of Greater London. The character of the area has been heavily influenced over the last half century by the creation of a number of large housing estates developed to re-house families from the war-damaged East End. The population, therefore, includes a significant number of people who were, as children, part of the mass evacuation from London during the Second World War, and/or were under the flight path of bombers during the Blitz.

The older people's mental health services include a CMHT, a psychiatric in-patient ward and a day hospital. Staff within the older people's CMHT include community psychiatric nurses (CPNs), occupational therapists (OTs) and social workers. They work in one of three localities within the borough, and each locality also has a Consultant in Old Age Psychiatry. In addition, there are support workers and OT technicians working across localities.

The services had seen major changes over the previous eight years due to the closure of the old psychiatric hospital and the disaggregation of mental health services from a community NHS Trust in order to merge with adjoining mental health services. Further changes included the closure of one of two psychiatric day hospitals and the formation of a multidisciplinary older people's CMHT. At around the same time, psychological services were re-configured such that psychologists were taken out of existing multidisciplinary teams into a borough-wide psychological therapies service alongside psychotherapists, art therapists and nurse therapists to provide a service for adults of all ages.

The older people's CMHT has become the single point of access for referrals over the age of 65 to the mental health service. The duty system within the older people's CMHT triages referrals to screening by an older people's CMHT worker, assessment by a psychiatrist in an out-patient clinic (for low-risk, non-urgent cases) or domiciliary visit (urgent/high risk), or assessment by the psychological therapies service.

Case studies

The cases referred to in this chapter are composites of case experiences over a number of years. This approach was taken to protect the anonymity and confidentiality of individuals and their families while drawing out common themes discussed within the services concerned.

Case 1: Mr K

Mr K was a 72-year-old married man with no history of mental health problems either personally or in his family. He was referred to older people's mental health services by his general practitioner (GP) who was concerned about Mr K's low mood, sense of hopelessness and lack of response to either antidepressant medication or input from the GP counsellor. Physically Mr K was well, aside from tablet-controlled diabetes and mild prostate problems. He had been prescribed Citalopram by his GP for the previous 10 weeks at a dose of 10mg.

Assessment

Mr K was initially assessed at the psychiatric out-patient clinic. His wife was also present, and corroborated his account of events. He described his symptoms as having begun after a sudden crisis of confidence while driving on holiday. He had been unable to continue the journey and his wife had driven them home. After this, Mr K experienced disturbed sleep. He gradually lost motivation to engage with activities of daily living and became progressively more withdrawn, effectively cutting himself off from his social circle and activities. He had lost his appetite and spent many hours worrying about what had gone wrong and what would become of him. He felt guilty for becoming a burden on his wife, and felt both ashamed and angry that he could not 'pull himself together' and 'snap out of it'. He described himself as 'useless' and 'pathetic'.

Diagnosis

The team psychiatrist diagnosed a mixed anxiety depressive state. Mr K's Citalopram was increased to 20mg once daily as the previous dose of 10mg was considered sub-therapeutic. It was planned that a CPN from the older people's CMHT would monitor medication over the next six weeks. There were no plans for wider service involvement, but an opportunity arose for short-term therapy with a junior psychiatrist who was keen to gain CBT experience.

Despite a therapeutic dose of medication and concurrent CBT therapy, Mr K's condition deteriorated. He was spending more time in bed, stopped drinking adequately and was expressing high levels of hopelessness. One weekend he developed an acute episode during which he appeared disorientated and confused with profound agitation and anxiety that did not respond to reassurance. During this he had a 'panic attack' when in the bathroom. Mrs K could hear her husband hyperventilating and feared that he was having a heart attack. The door was locked, and Mrs K could neither unlock it from outside nor focus Mr K's attention on her request that he unlock it. Mrs K called for an ambulance.

Mr K had managed to unlock the door before the paramedics entered the house, but both he and Mrs K were shaken by the experience. Mr K presented as short of breath, 'off-balance' and fearful of falling. Mrs K described him as having been 'muddled' all day. There were no clinical signs of heart attack, and both Mr and Mrs K were loath to attend A&E now that the immediate crisis appeared to have abated. The paramedics recommended that Mrs K contact the out-of-hours mental health number if Mr K's confusion or distress worsened. She called the next day. Mr K was voluntarily admitted to the older person's psychiatric in-patient unit for assessment. By the time of admission Mr K was disoriented in place and time and was unable to give a coherent history of events leading to admission. He underwent a thorough physical investigation including a full routine blood analysis including random and fasting glucose and urinalysis.

Standard psychometric assessments for the unit include the Geriatric Depression Scale (GDS-15; Yesavage *et al*. 1983) and the Mini-mental State Examination (MMSE; Folstein, Folstein and McHugh 1975). These were performed, but Mr K was poorly co-operative. MMSE revealed an initial score of 16/30 with deficits in multiple cognitive domains.

Intervention

Mr K's in-patient stay was brief. Based on the presentation and blood investigations revealing hyperglycaemia, Mr K's diabetic medication was re-instated, his blood glucose was monitored daily and his diet regulated. A review from the Consultant Physician visiting the ward confirmed the team's diagnosis of probable acute confusional state. Mr K's blood sugar quickly returned to the normal range with the above management.

Repeat cognitive assessment confirmed an improvement in MMSE score to 30/30 over the next week and a GDS indicated a score of 6/15. After a trial of successful home leave Mr K was discharged home.

A Care Programme Approach (CPA) discharge planning meeting agreed that Mr K be followed up by a CPN for medication monitoring. He was assessed for a place at the day hospital and started to attend one day a week. His wife transported him to and from the hospital, and he was a regular and punctual attendee. He took part in the activities on offer, and took to assisting the staff in helping with 'the old people'. Behaviourally, he seemed well at the day hospital, but when staff made comments to that effect he expressed concerns at his inability to 'get back to being his old self'. He described being unable to travel, not wanting to face former friends, lacking motivation at home and being unable to 'even start any of the little jobs that need to be done'.

Mr K was referred to psychological therapies on the basis that he was not progressing as far or as fast as he had the potential to do. In assessment Mr K described feeling 'different' to others and to his old self. He did not identify with any of his old friends nor with the day hospital attendees. Indeed, he was keen not to identify with them as he feared 'things getting as bad as they were for some of the poor folk on the ward'. Mr K described his shock at being admitted to a psychiatric unit and also his fear that he was on a 'downward slope' to dementia [the older person's psychiatric unit was a mixed ward for people with depression and dementia]. Mr K also feared that he was becoming alienated from his wife who could just 'get on with life' such that she was doing what had previously been 'his jobs' at home. The psychological formulation developed with Mr K highlighted his fears of 'getting old' and the psychological consequences of physical health problems in the context of previous good health. The impact of depression on his wife, and interpersonal maintaining factors were also discussed.

After considering whether he would prefer couple or individual work, Mr K undertook a 12-session individual cognitive behavioural intervention which included psychoeducation about, and coping strategies for, 'realistic' negative automatic thoughts (Moorey 1996). Self-defeating attitudes to ageing and mental health were addressed, and strategies were developed for practising 'compassionate responses' to his perceived failings. During the course of therapy Mr K was discharged from the day hospital and began attending a 'men's group' run by an OT from the older people's CMHT. By the end of therapy Mr K was reporting greater cheerfulness, less anxiety, greater levels of activity at home, a re-engagement with his previous social circle and greater empathy for people with mental health difficulties. He reported his wife as saying how pleased she was to 'have him back again', and the two of them were planning a number of short breaks now that he had started driving again. His scores on psychometric measures improved, and were no longer in the clinical range.

On-going support and evaluation

Mr K was followed up in the psychiatric out-patient clinic and given the option to reduce his antidepressant medication. He was wary of doing this, and chose to remain on the antidepressant. He had two post-therapy follow-up appointments with psychological therapies over the course of six months to review his progress using his 'well-being and recovery' plan (a Trust-wide initiative).

In Mr K's case the outcome was clear. He felt himself to be completely recovered and was also confident that he could take steps to address symptoms should they re-occur. He decided to leave the men's group to give more time for social activities with his wife, and they managed not only short breaks but also a three-week driving tour. Most satisfying from Mr K's point of view was again enjoying meeting friends, neighbours and acquaintances in the street. He was discharged from mental health services to the care of the GP.

Case 2: Mrs M

Mrs M had lost her husband within the last year after he had suffered a fatal heart attack. Mr and Mrs M had been married for 49 years and, on hearing news of Mr M's sudden death, the family had rallied round to support their mother. They had worried over the years about how she would cope 'if he went first', but they were relieved to find that she seemed to cope well, given the circumstances. However, in the weeks after the funeral, Mrs M's phone calls and requests for help became ever more frequent.

Levels of stress and distress rose on all sides and her family became exhausted trying to support her. Mrs M's elder daughter contacted the GP surgery and insisted that the GP 'do something', thus triggering the referral to the older people's CMHT.

Assessment approaches

Mrs M was initially seen by the duty CPN following an urgent referral from her GP. Mrs M was visibly shaking when the CPN arrived at her flat and was extremely tearful throughout the meeting. Mrs M described a range of somatic symptoms, and emotionally felt 'let down' and 'betrayed' by her family and her church who, she said, had 'abandoned' her after her husband's funeral. She said that she was terrified to stay in the flat on her own, and expressed a desire to move in with her younger daughter, who lived locally. She hoped that the CPN would be able to persuade the daughter of this idea, and stated that she would 'take all her tablets or something like that' if she needed to stay in her own flat. Mrs M shifted topic frequently and had difficulty focusing on questions, thus the CPN was only able to gather limited information on treatments and history (personal, family, physical and mental health).

The CPN returned to the older people's CMHT base with the intention of discussing Mrs M's case at the locality meeting that afternoon, but within 30 minutes of sitting at his desk, Mrs M had phoned him to say that she had told her younger daughter, Ann, that the CPN thought that she (Mrs M) should move into her (Ann's) house. While the CPN was still speaking with Mrs M on the phone, the CMHT receptionist came into the office to let the CPN know that there was a second caller for him. It was Ann, who was very angry and demanding to speak with the CPN. As family members are often involved in the provision of collateral history and in the treatment planning for clients in the service, it was not at all unusual for staff to make contact with relatives, and indeed for relatives to be the main point of contact in some cases. Given that he was at that moment speaking with Mrs M, the CPN took the opportunity to ask for her consent for him to speak with Ann. This permission was willingly granted, and the phone call ended with Mrs M repeating her desperate plea to get out of her flat.

Once Ann was speaking with the CPN she expressed her dissatisfaction and annoyance at the 'CPN's suggestion' that her mother move in with her. Ann was quickly pacified on hearing that the CPN had not made such a suggestion. She explained that her mother had a long history of 'playing' Ann and her siblings against each other to achieve the outcome she wanted, especially since they had left home and set up for themselves. The siblings had ended up in a number of arguments with each other over the years before they realised they had been 'set up' to clash by their mother. Their father had taken a backseat in discussion, and it was generally the elder daughter, Margaret, who ended up 'sorting things out'.

Ann was able to provide additional information about her mother who, she said, had 'fallen apart' after witnessing her husband's fatal heart attack. Initially, Mrs M had been very quiet and had spent long periods of time staring into space. She lost her appetite, lost interest in her appearance and stopped all her previous activities. She was regularly taking 'over the counter' sleep remedies in addition to Diazepam, but was unable to get to sleep at night. She moved between anger at her husband for 'leaving her to face things alone' and guilt that it was 'her fault' and that 'she should have gone first'.

Margaret had stayed with her mother in the weeks between her father's death and the funeral. When Margaret had needed to return to her own home and family after the funeral she had arranged a 'rota' with her siblings, nephews and nieces to visit Mrs M at meal-times to encourage her to eat. Despite these regular visits, Mrs M had taken to phoning family members she could find to answer the phone on the slightest pretext, or simply 'to hear a familiar voice'. Ann and Margaret felt increasingly drained and felt there was little option but to go along with their brother's suggestion that Mrs M move to a smaller and more comfortable accommodation in a retirement flat where there were others for company rather than be in the house on her own. An opportunity came up for a private purchase in a new development close to Mrs M's home. During the move Mrs M appeared to be picking up, but she deteriorated again once moved in. The phone calls to family members re-started. She made accusations that she had been forced to move when she had been quite happy in the family home. She said she had been robbed of her memories of time with her husband and complained constantly of loneliness.

The CPN had been acting as duty worker for the day, and had other cases that needed to be followed up. They therefore passed on their notes to the locality meeting.

Provisional diagnosis

Mrs M's case was discussed at the locality meeting and on the basis of the initial information the working diagnosis was depression in the context of bereavement, but that personality issues may play a significant role. As the only pharmacotherapy appeared to have been Diazepam it was agreed that it would be useful for Mrs M to be seen by the Consultant Psychiatrist to assess for antidepressant medication and also further assess the risk of self-harm, given Mrs M's threat to 'take all her tablets'. A domiciliary visit was arranged for the following afternoon.

When the Consultant Psychiatrist arrived, it was Mrs M's son who answered the door. He welcomed the visit and said that 'something needed to be done' as his mother was 'wreaking havoc' on all their lives. Mrs M was sitting in the front room, and said that she wanted her son to answer questions for her as she was 'too upset'. He gave a similar account of recent events as had been provided by Ann. In terms of history, he said that Mrs M had been born in the mid-1930s into a working-class family and was much younger than her four elder siblings. She had been evacuated during the Second World War, had never enjoyed school and had left at the minimum leaving age to work as a dressmaker. She had met her husband at a dance and, after a 'whirlwind romance', had married and had three children in close succession. He was not aware of any psychiatric history in the family, but said that Mrs M's physical health had always been poor, and she had often made reference to 'her nerves'. She had been on Valium (Diazepam) for a number of decades, as prescribed by the GP.

Mrs M had remained quiet throughout the interview, and had indeed seemed at times to be dozing. However, when he expressed his view that his mother 'needed to be in hospital' Mrs M became animated and disputed her son's implication that she 'was mad'. She accused others of 'not caring' and 'abandoning her'. She also expressed the view that 'in her day people respected their parents and would have done everything they could for them'. She made a direct plea to the psychiatrist for help, saying that she would be fine if only she could be back in her own home with her own belongings around her. She added no one understood how much pain she was in, described the anxiety attacks that she experienced when alone in the flat and her fear of shutting her eyes in case she saw her dead husband in front of her. Mrs M's son was unconcerned by his mother's outburst and distress saying that she had always known how to 'turn on the tears'. Mrs M repeated her threat to 'take all her tablets', but on further questioning the Consultant Psychiatrist established that it would be against her religious beliefs to take her own life.

Following the home visit the Consultant Psychiatrist dictated a letter for the GP excluding the diagnosis of abnormal or prolonged grief reaction, preferring a diagnosis of mild mixed anxiety depressive state noting, however, that there were significant features in relation to Mrs M's pre-morbid personality that most likely were contributing factors and indicators of poor prognosis. She noted the presence of Post-Traumatic Stress Disorder-like symptoms of hyper-arousal and flashbacks following the traumatic death of Mr M. She recommended the prescription of Escitalopram at 10mg in order to try to produce a rapid improvement and continued the use of Diazepam, 2mg taken only as needed up to twice a day, as this appeared helpful to Mrs M. She requested the allocation of a locality CPN and an assessment of activities of daily living by the OT. She also discussed the housing issue with the social worker who agreed to visit Mrs M to advise on options, given Mrs M's position of being able to self-fund.

Having drafted her assessment letter, the Consultant Psychiatrist received a call from Mrs M's daughter Margaret who said her world had been 'turned upside-down' by revelations made by her mother since her father's death. Her revelations had included Mrs M's father's alcoholism and intermittent physical violence, and his reaction to her when she returned from time away as an evacuee. She talked about a short-lived first marriage and her ambivalence towards Mr M whom she both loved for 'taking her on' and hated for his 'lack of passion' and 'covering up for her'. Hearing her mother's revelations had triggered childhood memories for Margaret of coming home from school to find her mother singing, whisky bottle in hand, and of unexplained absences when her mother went unexpectedly 'to stay with her sister'.

Margaret's account raised the likelihood that Mrs M had long-standing problems that had been contained/managed for decades by Mr M. The Consultant Psychiatrist added a referral to psychological therapies to her list of recommendations for intervention.

Intervention

As the planned intervention was implemented, Mrs M found reasons to dismiss all suggestions, yet repeatedly phoned staff to request help. She started to phone the allocated CPN to report all physical sensations that she attributed to medication side-effects. Initially the CPN, who also took on the role of CPA care co-ordinator, listened to her concerns and provided reassurance, but the frequency of calls increased to the extent that he started to request that reception tell her that he was out, and also ignored some of her requests to call urgently. The team manager became involved due to concern that ignoring 'urgent' calls would be criticised should there be a serious untoward incident requiring investigation.

The OT was unable to complete her assessment. Mrs M had refused to co-operate saying that she 'had always looked after her home and would still be able to if she wanted, but she did not wish to carry on living in the flat'. Provision of a careline failed to provide any reassurance for Mrs M. Indeed both the family and call-centre requested that it be removed as Mrs M was making inappropriate call-outs at all times of the day and night. Mrs M did not wish to hear about social and occupational activities as 'it was her family that she needed'.

The social worker tried to discuss housing options with Mrs M, but she maintained that now her home had been sold, the only option was to live with one of her children, who 'owed it to her' to support her after all the years that she had dedicated to looking after them. Her children, however, were all very firm with the social worker that it was not an option for Mrs M to live with any of them, but were unwilling to say this directly to her for fear of 'making things worse'.

Mrs M had seen the psychologist for assessment and had turned down the offer of any individual work unless it could be in the flat. Her presentation was such that it seemed unlikely that she would be able to engage with a 'symptom oriented' CBT, and at the time there were no psychological therapists able to provide home visits for either bereavement or psychodynamic work. The family rejected 'family therapy' in the systemic clinic but were willing to attend a 'family meeting'.

During the early involvement of the older people's CMHT, Mrs M appeared to further 'unravel' rather than stabilise or improve. The family had taken the opportunity to withdraw to a certain extent and Mrs M added CMHT members to her list of people to call when lonely or agitated in her flat. She would be in tears and keen to have physical contact with any visitors. The frequency and intensity of threats of self-harm increased, but she did not act on any of them. Mrs M's situation was raised every week at the locality referrals meeting, and it was decided to call an early CPA meeting.

In advance of the CPA meeting, there were a number of discussions between various team members. The team discussed admission to the in-patient unit, but anticipated that this would be strongly opposed by Mrs M and both her daughters. In addition, experience from a similar case had been that while admission provided temporary respite for the family, there was no behavioural change on return home. There were different opinions within the team over the extent to which Mrs M was 'purposefully manipulative' and 'attention seeking', and the extent to which she should be reassured or told not to call. The psychologist proposed that the team use a dialectic behaviour therapy type approach, as used in the treatment of borderline personality disorders. In this, the main strategies are the validation of emotions while maintaining strict behavioural boundaries. Although some team members expressed an interest, the majority were averse to the idea. A formal diagnosis of personality disorder had not been made and staff felt that the intervention was beyond their remit. They feared that risk may not be appropriately managed and the required level of input was beyond the capacity of what they could provide.

The CPA review was attended by Mrs M and all her children, even though relations between them and their mother were now very poor. During the meeting, the issue of living accommodation was addressed directly for the first time with all parties present. Mrs M was able to describe how terrified she felt when left alone, and her children were each able to say why they were unable to accommodate their mother. As expected, all members of the family continued to object strongly to in-patient admission being considered. Mrs M (reluctantly) agreed to a respite stay in residential care, and the family were pleased. The specialist personality disorder service was also mentioned, and it was agreed to make a referral on the basis of presenting behaviours.

On-going support and evaluation

Although Mrs M reported barely tolerating her respite stay, staff in the home described her as being 'fine, if a little demanding'. The family were happy with their mother's respite stay. Assessment by the personality disorders service did not open up any new options and indeed a recommendation was made for a 'care home'. The family agreed to investigate possible residential settings, in discussion with the social worker, and once this decision had been made there was greater stability in the system. Mrs M continued to call the older people's CMHT and family members with great regularity, but staff felt less 'bombarded' now that 'there was an end in sight' and Mrs M's level of distress and pleading had subsided. Mrs M continued to express reluctance over the proposed move but assented to visits and expressed opinions on 'likes' as well as 'dislikes'. There were considerable discussions within the team as a number of ethical issues were raised including the conflict of the rights of the individual versus the right of family not to provide care, and competence to consent in a cognitively intact but emotionally distressed individual. As Mrs M was again self-funding, the choices available were greater than if she required a funded placement. There was no need for her to fulfil the criteria for residential or nursing need. Although the family had expressed concern over the cost of accommodation they were keen to have some resolution to this challenging episode of their lives.

Once a residential bed was available, the older people's CMHT staff advised the family on the importance of Mrs M taking personal mementoes and familiar furniture with her into residential care. They also briefed the home manager on medication management for Mrs M, the importance of making her feel welcome and of having a good relationship with her allocated key worker. To the surprise of the older people's CMHT staff, Mrs M settled well and she was discharged from the older people's CMHT six weeks after she moved.

After a successful 'honeymoon period', Mrs M re-started making frequent phone calls to the family; who in turn re-contacted the older people's CMHT. The CPN made a visit to review medication and circumstances. It transpired that a worker with whom Mrs M had formed a particularly close bond had moved away at the same time as the home manager was on annual leave. The situation improved when the home manager returned, but remained fragile.

Discussion and conclusion

The two case studies share a diagnosis of mixed anxiety depressive states. The first case, Mr K, illustrates the way in which anxiety symptoms contribute to a spiral of inter-acting physical decline and mood disturbance, especially in the context of negative attitudes to age and ageing. The second case, Mrs M, highlights the devastating impact of loneliness, and the anxiety that can be unleashed as a consequence of the breaking of emotional bonds.

Team decision making

Issues of perceived health, attitudes to age, and loneliness are closely aligned to prevailing themes in the gerontological literature, but receive little consideration in guidance for treatment of anxiety and depression by mental health teams. Decisions made by, and within, the team are often on the basis of prior experience rather than the 'evidence base', due to the lack of pertinent clinical/intervention literature. An advantage of a dedicated CMHT for older people, rather than integrated provision for people of all ages, is the accumulated and shared knowledge of common presentations in later life. For example, given that poor physical health is a significant risk factor for those developing either a depression or a mixed state (Vink *et al.* 2009), it is important to distinguish between understandable and realistic concerns about physical health and a somatic preoccupation which forms part of a distinct psychiatric condition. Awareness of typical symptom profiles in older cohorts aids this kind of decision-making within the team.

Shared knowledge of common age-specific and cohort-specific issues assists with the development of care plans that target the needs of the individual rather than 'treating the diagnosis'. For example, Mr K expressed the 'age specific' fear of falling. Fear of falling is known to have a limiting effect on activity which, in turn, is associated with a lowering of mood.

Mrs M provides an example of a cohort-specific issue, given her experience of being a wartime evacuee. The evacuation of British children during the Second World War has resulted in a lower incidence of secure attachment styles compared with those who were not evacuated, with a corresponding increase in fearful styles (Rusby and Tasker 2008). Mrs M's disrupted attachments in childhood are likely to have coloured subsequent relationships and understanding of these influenced the older people's CMHT decision-making. The long-term impact of the Second World War may also explain some of the local variations in depressive symptoms in the oldest old (Copeland *et al*. 2004).

Team decisions are also influenced by organisational factors and the availability of services. For example, admissions policy to the in-patient ward has changed with the reduction in bed numbers and the formation of a Home Treatment Team, which now acts as 'gatekeeper' for the wards. 'Crisis services' that cover the over 65s are not the norm across England. Indeed, in a survey in 2006 of 79 English Trusts providing acute mental health services and at least one crisis resolution team, only one in six areas regularly provided crisis services to older people (Cooper *et al*. 2007). This finding is in keeping with the broad acknowledgement from the Department of Health that older people have tended not to benefit as much as younger people in service modernisation (Department of Health 2005). The '*Everybody's Business*' initiative was intended to assist service providers in service development and modernisation (Department of Health and Care Service Improvement Partnership 2005). The dedicated website includes links to a range of service development guidelines (www.everybodysbusiness.org.uk; accessed 8 February 2010) aimed at ensuring non-discriminatory and inclusive services.

Mrs M's case demonstrates the way in which issues of resources and consent influence the care pathway. If Mrs M were not self-funding and if she had not assented to visit homes then there would have been debate with adult protection over the appropriateness, or otherwise, of placement. Protracted funding negotiations may have arisen between the trust and local authority. Had her mental state worsened further and if she refused voluntary admission to hospital, then admission under the *Mental Health Act* (1983) would have been considered.

A risk to the team is the pervasive influence of negative attitudes to ageing that are so common in the population served, and may serve to lower the expectations of recovery. Working exclusively within mental health precludes contact with 'successful agers' and the beliefs that characterise them. Tools such as Laidlaw and colleagues' 'Attitudes of Ageing' scale provide a useful insight into personal beliefs about ageing, for both staff and clients (Laidlaw *et al*. 2007).

Family involvement

In contrast to services for working age adults, contact with the families of referred clients is often the norm rather than an exception in mental health services for older people. This is perhaps an artefact from the time when old age psychiatry was in its infancy, and the population was characterised by a high level of frailty-related dependence on others. As life-expectancy, and more importantly the number of 'healthy' years, has increased, family involvement may not always be welcomed by referred clients. Both case studies raise issues of the need to balance client confidentiality and communication with family carers.

Access to psychological therapies

There is a long-standing stereotype of a lack of 'psychological mindedness' on the part of the older person themselves, which has led to an assumption that older people are neither willing nor 'suitable' to engage with psychotherapeutic work. While it is not unusual for the current cohort of older people to have little knowledge of psychological therapies, this does not necessarily equate to resistance to the idea. Indeed, in a study of preferences for treatment for depression psychological approaches were often preferred to pharmacological options (Landreville *et al.* 2001).

Therapist services have been a scarce resource in mental health care. The Improving Access to Psychological Therapies (IAPT) initiative aims to increase the number of trained (CBT) therapists available to the NHS. The IAPT initiative is for people of all ages (Improving Access to Psychological Therapies 2009), and has a particular focus on anxiety and depression. However, while emphasising the importance of equity on the grounds of factors such as age, culture and ethnicity, the therapist training curriculum makes no reference to pertinent issues for older generations, such as cohort issues, life-span development, physical health or bereavement.

Despite the strong evidence base for CBT for younger people, and an evidence for its effectiveness in later life, CBT is little or no better than other psychotherapeutic approaches for late-life depression. There is a need for development work to enhance the effectiveness of CBT with older people. Mr K's comment that CBT taught him 'what I know already – it's my fault for not thinking more positively' is pertinent here. It gives insight into a common misapprehension of the 'core message' of CBT and the demoralising impact that 'rational response training' can have. 'Third wave' CBT approaches, including process-focused interventions and compassionate mind training, may prove to be of particular benefit to current cohorts of older people who place a high value on being 'useful'. Similarly, transdiagnostic approaches to CBT should be considered for use with older cohorts given the multiplicity of presenting problems.

Limitations

Anxiety and depression in later life is a wide-ranging topic, and we have necessarily narrowed our focus for this chapter, choosing to illustrate 'late-onset' depression in adults living in their own homes. Issues relating to 'graduates' of adult mental health have not been discussed, but include the influence of past treatment and of previous relationships with staff, on current presentation. Anxiety and depression in people with cognitive impairments have not been considered; nor has the overlapping symptomatology of chronic lung conditions or heart disorders with anxiety states; nor the similarities in symptoms between depression and a range of physical disorders, such as thyroid difficulties.

Conclusions

Policy documents on the treatment of anxiety and depression provide only limited guidance for older people's CMHT staff, given the absence of reference to age or ageing. Decision-making by teams is therefore heavily influenced by knowledge of common themes and by previous experience. There is a need for new interventions to be developed that address key factors in late-life anxiety and depression.

References

Age Concern and the Mental Health Foundation (2007) *Improving services and support for older people with mental health problems. The second report from the UK inquiry into mental health and well-being in later life*, London: Age Concern and the Mental Health Foundation. Available: www.mhilli.org/documents/Inquiryfinalreport-fullreport.pdf (accessed 4 February 2010).

Astrom, M. (1996) 'Generalized Anxiety Disorder in stroke patients', *Stroke*, 27: 270–75.

Ayers, C., Sorrell, J., Thorp, S. and Wetherell, J. (2007) 'Evidence-based psychological treatments for late-life anxiety', *Psychology and Aging*, 22: 8–17.

Baldwin, D.S., Anderson, I.M., Nutt, D.J., Bandelow, B., Bond, A., Davidson, J.R.T., den Boer, J.A., Fineberg, N.A., Knapp, M., Scott, J. and Wittchen, H.-U. (2005) 'Evidence based guidelines for the pharmacological treatment of anxiety disorder: recommendations from the British Association for Psychopharmacology', *Journal of Psychopharmacology*, 19: 567–96.

Bryant, C., Jackson, H. and Ames, D. (2008) 'The prevalence of anxiety in older adults: methodological issues and a review of the literature', *Journal of Affective Disorders*, 109: 233–50.

Cooper, C., Regan, C., Tandy, A., Johnson, S. and Livingston, G. (2007) 'Acute mental health care for older people by crisis resolution teams in England', *International Journal of Geriatric Psychiatry*, 22: 263–65.

Copeland, J.R.M., Beekman, A.T.F., Braam, A.W., Dewey, M.E., Delespaul, P., Fuhrer, R., Hooijer, C., Lawlor, B.A., Kivela, S.-L., Lobo, A., Magnusson, H., Mann, A.H., Meller, I., Prince, M.J., Reischies, F., Roelands, M., Skoog, I., Turrina, C., deVries, M.W. and Wilson, K.C.M. (2004) 'Depression among older people in Europe: the EURODEP studies', *World Psychiatry*, 3: 45–49.

Department of Health (2001) *National Service Framework for Older People: Modern Standards and Service Models*, London: Department of Health.

——(2005) *Securing better mental health for older adults*, London: Department of Health.

Department of Health and Care Service Improvement Partnership (2005) *Everybody's Business: Integrated Mental Health Services for Older Adults: a service development guide*, London: Department of Health.

Flint, A. (2005) 'Generalised anxiety disorders in elderly patients: epidemiology, diagnosis and treatment options', *Drugs and Aging*, 22: 101–14.

Folstein, M.F., Folstein, S. and McHugh, P. (1975) 'Mini-mental State: a practical method for grading the cognitive state of patients for the clinician', *Journal of Psychiatric Research*, 12: 189–98.

Improving Access to Psychological Therapies (2009) *Older People: Positive Practice Guide*, London: Department of Health.

Kvaal, K., McDougall, F.A., Brayne, C., Matthews, F.E. and Dewey, M.C. (2008) 'Co-occurrence of anxiety and depression in a community sample of older people: results from the MRC CFAS', *International Journal of Geriatric Psychiatry*, 23: 229–37.

Laidlaw, K., Power, M.J., Schmidt, S. and the WHOQOL-OLD group (2007) 'The Attitudes to Ageing questionnaire (AAQ): development and psychometric properties', *International Journal of Geriatric Psychiatry*, 22: 367–79.

Landreville, P., Landry, J., Baillargeon, L., Guerette, A. and Matteau, E. (2001) 'Older adults' acceptance of psychological and pharmacological treatments for depression', *Journals of Gerontology: Psychological Sciences*, 50B: 285–91.

Mahoney, R., Regan, C., Katona, C. and Livingston, G. (2005) 'Anxiety and depression in family caregivers of people with Alzheimer's disease', *American Journal of Geriatric Psychiatry*, 13: 795–801.

Montgomery, S., Chatamra, K., Pauer, L., Whalen, E. and Baldinetti, F. (2008) 'Efficacy and safety of pregabalin in elderly people with generalized anxiety disorder', *British Journal of Psychiatry*, 193: 389–94.

Moorey, S. (1996) 'When bad things happen to rational people: Cognitive therapy in adverse life circumstances', in P. Salkovskis (ed.), *Frontiers of cognitive therapy*, New York: Guilford Press.

Mukai, Y. and Tampi, R. (2009) 'Treatment of depression in the elderly: a review of the recent literature on the efficacy of single-versus dual-action antidepressants', *Clinical Therapeutics*, 31: 945–61.

National Collaborating Centre for Mental Health (2007) *Depression: management of depression in primary and secondary care – NICE guidance*, London: National Institute for Health and Clinical Excellence. Available: www.nice.org.uk/cg023 (accessed 8 February 2010).

National Collaborating Centre for Primary Care (2007) *Anxiety: management of anxiety (panic disorder, with or without agoraphobia, and generalized anxiety disorder) in adults in primary, secondary and community care*, London: National Institute for Health and Clinical Excellence. Available: www.nice.org.uk/cg022 (accessed 8 February 2010).

Rusby, J.S.M. and Tasker, F. (2008) 'Childhood temporary separation: long-term effects of the British evacuation of children during World War II on older adults' attachment styles', *Attachment & Human Development*, 10: 207–21.

Scogin, F., Welsh, D., Hanson, A., Stump, J. and Coates, A. (2005) 'Evidence based psychotherapies for depression in older adults', *Clinical Psychology: Science and Practice*, 12: 222–37.

Vink, D., Aartsen, M. and Schoevers, R. (2008) 'Risk factors for anxiety and depression in the elderly: a review', *Journal of Affective Disorders*, 106: 29–44.

Vink, D., Aartsen, M.J., Camijs, H., Heymans, M.J., Penninx, B.W.J.H., Stek, M.L., Deeg, D.J.H. and Beekman, A.T.F. (2009) 'Onset of anxiety and depression in the aging population: comparison of risk factors in a 9 year prospective study', *American Journal of Geriatric Psychiatry*, 17: 642–52.

Yesavage, J.A., Brink, T.L., Lum, O., Huang, V., Adey, M.B> and Leirer, V.O. (1983) 'Development and validation of a geriatric depression screening scale: A preliminary report', *Journal of Psychiatric Research*, 17: 37–49.

5 Ageing and psychosis

Susan Mary Benbow, Julie Grainger, Moganeswari Grizzell and Faye Pemberton

Key messages

- Psychosis in older adults is uncommon.
- The question of if (and when) people who grow old with an established psychotic illness should transfer from the general adult to older adult mental health service can be contentious.
- In order to establish a therapeutic alliance a person-centred approach to assessment and treatment is essential.
- Good communication with the service user and their family and between team members and other involved agencies is key to co-ordinating a treatment plan.
- Holistic treatment plans will address physical, psychological and social aspects of care.

Introduction

Definition of the condition

The classification of psychotic disorders in later life remains an area which lacks clarity. The terms late-onset (or very-late-onset) schizophrenia and paraphrenia are both sometimes used for people who develop a new psychotic illness in later life. The International Late-Onset Schizophrenia Group in 1998 (Howard *et al.* 2000) produced a consensus statement which recognised late-onset schizophrenia (with onset after the age of 40 years) and very-late-onset schizophrenia-like psychosis (with onset after the age of 60 years). The Group regarded typical-onset schizophrenia as having an age of onset between 15 and 40 years. The group of disorders described by the term very-late-onset schizophrenia-like psychosis is sometimes still called paraphrenia by practising old age psychiatrists.

The International Classification of Diseases (ICD)-10 classifies the paraphrenias as persistent delusional disorders (F22.0) (World Health Organization 2007). ICD-10 requires delusions to be the only, or the most prominent, feature of the clinical presentation and to have been present for at least three months. It describes the disorders as 'persistent and sometimes lifelong' and notes that persistent auditory hallucinations or evidence of organic brain disease are incompatible with the diagnosis.

In practice old age psychiatrists often use late-onset schizophrenia to describe illnesses which start in later life (aged over 60 or 65) but would fulfil diagnostic criteria for schizophrenia, and paraphrenia to describe psychosis with onset in later life with prominent delusions which would not fulfil strict diagnostic criteria for schizophrenia. In this chapter, for simplicity, this is the terminology which will be used.

There is a third group of older adults with psychosis to consider: namely, those who developed a schizophrenic illness later in life and have grown old with persisting illness.

Demographics and prevalence

Population studies suggest that psychosis is uncommon in older adults with a prevalence of less than 3 percent, but becomes more common with greater age (Howard *et al.* 2000). Ostling and Skoog (2002) found an increased three-year incidence of dementia in a population of Swedish 85-year-olds with hallucinations, delusions and paranoid ideation.

Female gender is associated with later age of onset and in later life the ratio of women to men may be as high as 8:1 (Eyler Zorrilla and Jeste 2002). Cohen *et al.* (2004) found a significantly greater prevalence of paranoid ideation or psychotic symptoms amongst black elders compared with their white counterparts in an urban population.

Synthesis of key literature

Later onset of illness has been said to be linked with a milder illness, better preserved personality, better outcome and a reduced risk of schizophrenia in first-degree relatives than amongst people with a younger age of onset (Howard *et al.* 1997). Almeida *et al.* (1995a) investigated risk factors and found marked increases in hearing impairment, the likelihood of living alone and the likelihood of being rated as socially isolated in the patient group. They also found an increase in soft neurological signs suggesting that older adults who develop a late-onset psychosis might be more likely to have underlying organic brain disease even if this is not clinically apparent.

People who have a late-onset schizophrenia are more likely than their younger counterparts to have visual, tactile and olfactory hallucinations, but are much less likely to have formal thought disorder, negative symptoms and affective blunting. Almeida *et al.* (1995b) reported that a wide range of delusions occurred in a group they studied who were described as having 'late paraphrenia' (over 80 percent were persecutory). They also commonly had auditory hallucinations (almost 80 percent). Formal thought disorder was very uncommon, and none of their group had catatonic symptoms or inappropriate affect. They described the delusions and hallucinations as 'usually so exuberant as to dominate ... [the] clinical picture'.

Treatment of psychosis in older adults often involves the use of anti-psychotic drugs, but it is important to consider pharmacological and non-pharmacological approaches. It may be helpful to divide the latter into psychological and social treatments. Karim and Byrne (2005) regard the usefulness of drug treatments as well-established, and state that atypical anti-psychotics are 'more suitable' for older adults.

There is a lack of research on applying treatments used with younger adults with older people with psychosis.

Policy considerations

Key policy drivers

The important policy documents to be considered in relation to services for people with a psychosis in late life are the *National Service Frameworks (NSFs) for Mental Health* (Department of Health 1999) and *Older People* (Department of Health 2001). Although the NSF for Mental Health initially applied to people of working age, it is now understood to apply across the age range. The NSF for Older People includes a specific Standard addressing the mental health of older people, but perhaps more importantly addresses mental health in relation to other areas of older people's physical health care. *Everybody's Business* (Department of Health and Care Services Improvement Partnership 2005) has been published since the *NSF for Older People* (Department of Health 2001) and gives a more detailed template for older people's mental health services. A professional document, which is also relevant, is the Faculty of Old Age Psychiatry (2006) publication, *Raising the Standard*.

An important issue for people with a psychotic illness in later life is the question of whether their care is more appropriately provided by general adult or older adult services and there are documents which consider this dilemma. *Links not boundaries* is a recently published report from the Royal College of Psychiatrists (2009), which gives recommendations about service transitions as people grow older. A working group at the Royal College of Psychiatrists (2004) previously set out some general principles relating to this issue. They stated that the service with the greatest expertise in relation to the care needs of a particular individual should take responsibility for their care and that service users should always receive the service most appropriate to their needs. However, they also argue that continuity of care should take precedence over automatic referral to older adult services in respect of physically well people without dementia over the age of 65 years (which would include people who are growing older with an established psychotic illness). The working group regarded the age of 65 as a useful service boundary for people who present for the first time with a psychiatric disorder.

This transition issue links with concern about what has been called 'age equality', an issue raised by concerns that there is inequality in health care for older people. The *UK Inquiry into Mental Health and Well-Being in Later Life* flagged up concerns about age discrimination in the health care of older adults in its first report (Age Concern and the Mental Health Foundation 2006). Care Services Improvement Partnership (2007) has issued a guidance note in response to debate about this area, reiterating a point which might seem to be uncontroversial and self-evident, that services should be needs-based rather than age-based.

Another area of some controversy has been the relationship between the Single Assessment Process (Department of Health 2002) and the Care Programme Approach (CPA) (Department of Health 2008), and how this comes into play when people cross the boundary between younger and older adult services.

Applying principles

About our team

Wolverhampton was awarded city status on 1 January 2001 and lies 13 miles to the north-west of Birmingham. It is sometimes described as the capital of the Black Country, and is surrounded by countryside to the north-west and south-west. The resident population of the Wolverhampton Metropolitan Borough is approximately 250,000: in broad figures 23,000 residents are aged 65–74 years and 19,000 aged over 75. Predictions are that the population profile is likely to show little change up until 2016. The catchment population for acute services is larger than this, since the specialist services in Wolverhampton are used by people from surrounding towns and villages.

The psychiatric service is provided in three sectors, each of which has a community mental health team (CMHT) and one (or two in the case of the south-west sector) consultant psychiatrist(s). In-patient beds for older adults are provided in a mental health unit across the city from the acute hospital services. There are some city-wide older adult mental health services, including an Asian Link Service, an African-Caribbean Link Service, a Memory Clinic, an Older Adult Liaison Service and an Older Adult Home Treatment Team. In the sector contributing here, the CMHT is based in a joint social services/ health resource centre where day care, respite care and long-term residential care is also provided.

Case studies

The cases described as AB and CD are based on an amalgam of experiences with people working with the team and do not describe individual service users. The team thanks the service users and families whose experiences have contributed to these case studies, and our team colleagues who worked with them alongside us.

Case study 1: Mrs AB

AB was a 66-year-old divorced woman under the care of the general psychiatry service. She had been diagnosed with paranoid schizophrenia and had been in contact with services for several decades and through various changes of community psychiatric nurse and psychiatrist. She had a history of several admissions to hospital, usually as a detained patient under the *Mental Health Act* (1983). When she complied with treatment she would function well, but would still have no insight into her illness, saying that the people who had been bothering her had gone away. She lived alone in a small flat with regular visits from her daughter and grand-daughter, and was interested in sewing and knitting. She was maintained on regular depot anti-psychotic injections, given by her general adult community nurse. Her physical health was generally good, although she was on medication for high blood pressure, diabetes and arthritis.

Six months before her referral to the older people's mental health service she discontinued her depot injections against advice and over the next few months gradually became unwell, expressing ideas that people were coming into the house, taking her things without her consent and making a mess in the kitchen. Her sleep became disturbed and she lost weight, saying she couldn't cook any more as people were using her kitchen and making a mess while she was asleep or out of the house. She told her daughter that she thought 'druggies' were behind it, a view she had expressed during previous episodes, and took to haranguing passers-by in the street as she believed they were selling drugs to the people who were interfering in her life. Matters came to a head after she assaulted a businessman who had parked his car down the road, believing that he was a drug dealer, and the police were called.

After a *Mental Health Act* (1983) assessment AB was admitted on a Section 3 to an old age psychiatry ward, because there were no general psychiatry beds and, since she was over the age of 65, the professionals involved felt that her care would best be transferred to older people's services.

Assessment approaches

An early issue was whether it had been appropriate to transfer AB's care in an emergency to a team which had no prior knowledge of her, when she had established relationships with a general psychiatrist and a community nurse in the general adult CMHT. This led to some difficulties as AB was angry that she had to get to know new people as well as being angry about her admission, with which she strongly disagreed.

Thus her assessment was carried out by a team new to her and her circumstances, which had not been involved in the decision to admit her under the *Mental Health Act* (1983). An important part of her assessment was to get as much information as possible about her, including obtaining old psychiatric and medical notes relating to her treatment, which were scrutinised in detail in order to learn how she had responded to various treatments in the past. The diagnosis was not in doubt as she had previously expressed the same ideas when she had been ill, and she continued to have auditory hallucinations and express delusional beliefs on the ward. It was also clear that at no stage in the past had she gained insight into her illness: she had never accepted that she had a mental illness. She appealed against her Section and a Tribunal was due to be held two months after her admission, by which time she had improved, had been taken off her Section and had opted to remain an in-patient. She had assaulted someone prior to admission, so ward staff were concerned that she had demonstrated unpredictability in the past and carried out a risk assessment, to assess the risk to other patients, visitors and staff as part of the CPA process. This had to be regularly updated and reviewed as she soon started to go on organised trips off the ward with an occupational therapist, although she always came back without demur.

While on the ward, staff used Roper's model for needs assessment and care planning (Roper, Logan and Tierney 1981). This offers an individualised holistic approach based on 12 components of an individual's activities of living, such as maintaining a safe environment and communicating.

The team aimed to maintain or restore AB's abilities, and in this the occupational therapist had a key role, closely linked with ward nursing staff. In order to match AB's abilities with the demands of her occupations and environment, the team needed to establish a collaborative relationship with her. It is important to note that both the maintenance and improvement to functional ability takes place within the context of that person's illness or disability (Creek 2003); therefore, the occupational therapist and other team members carry out therapeutic interventions whilst a service user is still experiencing symptoms of their illness. As a team, we believe that this work should start as soon as possible after admission and, despite her frustration with being in hospital, AB soon engaged with the team as she hoped to go home at the earliest possible opportunity.

Initially, the occupational therapist collected as much information as possible and spoke with her informally to establish rapport. At the initial assessment AB gave consent for occupational therapy treatment and intervention: 'clients shall be given sufficient information to enable them to give informed consent about their health and social care' (College of Occupational Therapists 2005). In collaboration and negotiation with AB, she started to identify difficulties, together with goals that AB wished to achieve (Sumsion 2000). The involvement of service users within the initial assessment is essential as it recognises that they are the 'experts' on their own problems, and at the centre of decision-making. It encourages the service user to be autonomous and take control, as well as ensuring that the service user is engaged in the creation and direction of therapeutic activity. These elements are believed to be associated with improved outcomes, satisfaction and compliance (Hong *et al.* 2000). This is the approach which was followed with AB.

At first, AB felt angry about being with the older adult service and highlighted differences within the service which she felt were detrimental to her care. She was at that time difficult to engage with, as she showed some hostility and suspicion towards staff managing her care. However, as a team, it was felt important to get to know AB to ascertain her needs, including what was purposeful to her. Our approach is client centred and embodies a service user/therapist partnership. The occupational therapist works to empower the service user to engage in functional activities and achieve necessary roles in various environments. Intervention is usually more effective when the service user is fully engaged (Sumsion 2000).

The team decided that the best way to assess AB's functional abilities was through observation of functioning and activity analysis. Analysis provides information of how activities contribute to the balance between skills in daily living, productivity and leisure, and motivate a person to organise routines into behavioural patterns and roles (Johnson 1996). It is believed that by using standardised assessments professionals are in danger of practising with a reductionist approach and this is highlighted when decisions are made about an older person's competence on the basis of a single assessment: this has the potential for a person to be treated as a 'thing' rather than an individual (McCormack 2004). In AB's case, poor literacy skills may have given an inaccurate picture of current abilities. As an occupational therapy department the focus was on completing appropriate functional assessments over a period of time, concentrating on her individual strengths. AB had been living at home independently, although latterly with difficulty, prior to admission into in-patient care. It was discovered she had a great interest in cooking and baking but was impeded by her poor reading and writing skills, as she was unable to read recipes and instructions. She expressed an interest in sewing and other creative activities. It was also important to her to be able to complete her own laundry.

Drug treatment was an important part of AB's management, alongside psychological, occupational and social aspects of treatment throughout her admission and subsequently. Negotiating the medication treatment plan was a challenge as AB had no insight into her illness and the old notes suggested that she had never fully gained insight. Part of the psychological management was to establish a therapeutic relationship with AB and to establish a way of talking with her about her experiences. A family meeting was offered but AB's daughter refused: perhaps she was so relieved to have her mother in hospital that she opted not to engage and instead to take a break.

One major difficulty in terms of recommending drug treatment was that it was difficult to find out how much of a recovery AB had made between her previous acute episodes of illness. This demonstrated that mental health staff are much better at recording details of illness than details of health and level of recovery and function during periods of relative wellness. When staff who had cared for her previously were approached, they all had differing views on this matter. Her daughter felt that when well, her mother had no signs or symptoms of psychotic illness. It was difficult for a team new to AB to reconcile these differing viewpoints.

AB's transfer into the old age psychiatry service also involved a change of social worker and this gave the new social worker the chance to carry out a re-assessment of her needs and a carer's assessment with her daughter. The latter offered an opportunity to engage AB's family in her assessment and subsequent treatment. Since AB lacked insight, consent was an issue throughout her treatment. She was able to understand details of drug treatments, side-effects and potential benefits but did not admit that she was ill, although she could describe her history of contact with mental health services. She had strong views about which medications were suitable for her, whilst simultaneously denying that she really needed treatment.

Communication during the admission centred on ward team meetings. It is our usual practice to encourage patients to be in the room with staff, provided they feel comfortable to be so, throughout the discussion about their progress and treatment, and to engage actively in the discussion and debate. Occupational therapy and nursing staff use joint records but currently social care uses separate records and, unfortunately, health and social care computers don't talk to each other: this makes the team meetings an important and necessary opportunity for all disciplines to meet and exchange ideas and information. CPA meetings are held as part of ward team meetings and, since AB was already registered for CPA, this continued.

Intervention

After reviewing her past history, AB was prescribed an oral anti-psychotic which she had found helpful before, and later, with her agreement, started on a depot anti-psychotic which she had previously taken with evidence of response. Despite continuing to protest that she was not ill and did not need treatment, she complied with medication and began to express fewer delusional ideas. She also started to accept her new psychiatrist and other team members, and to say who she would like to follow her up after discharge.

During her acute illness, she had failed to comply with treatment for her physical conditions so part of her management involved attending to her physical health, including explaining to her why she needed drugs in order to get her diabetes and blood pressure back under control.

As she settled on the ward, AB became calmer and more relaxed, and established relationships with team members. AB and her family were also referred for behavioural family therapy to look at coping strategies for the future and family education. The main issue on the ward was trust. She had two key nurses who worked to build up trust with AB during this period.

During her admission AB engaged in group activities in the occupational therapy department whilst on the ward, as well as several individual activities. These included baking, art, pottery, gardening, reminiscence and, latterly, community outings. She appeared to find engaging within group situations more difficult, at times becoming hostile to either staff or other service users mainly due to misinterpretation of what others said or her delusional thoughts. When she did engage in activities, she demonstrated great skill and with verbal instruction she was able to produce baked products and crafts to high standards, which appeared to please her. Our philosophy is that throughout this process team members should respect the service users' values and listen to them, and that treatment plans should be individualised. Each service user has a unique personality, occupational needs, social and family context and, more importantly, life history. Sometimes interventions may need to be adapted to meet needs, to enable choice and to be person-centred (Sumsion 2000, Creek 2003): as AB found group environments difficult at times, one-to-one intervention was used. AB appeared to enjoy the attention of a one-to-one session; at times she would become distracted by negative thoughts, but could be quickly re-engaged by talking with her about her achievements, about close family members and the continuation of the activity. It was important to her to continue her domestic activities of daily living. She was able to complete her own laundry, facilitated by the occupational therapy department on a regular basis. This continued throughout her admission, along with the maintenance of other daily living skills. AB became particularly hostile towards one member of the team: she was suspicious and paranoid about written information, particularly when it was written in her presence. She had noted on several occasions that one member of the team was writing notes. When this became an issue, the occupational therapist stopped making notes in her presence and withdrew from meetings at AB's request.

The team needs to ensure that older people are involved in any pre-discharge decisions made and therapists need to justify clinically the grounds for a home visit and how it will contribute to improving a person's quality of life (Atwal *et al.* 2008). AB was taken on an occupational therapy home visit to assess and monitor her functional abilities, mental state and behaviour, and to help determine what she needed by way of support following discharge. Whilst there she spoke about her perceived difficulties with neighbours, believing them to be responsible for her difficulties prior to assessment. During the visit AB talked at length about moving to a different location and decided she would pursue this after discharge – the social worker was alerted to the need to pursue the possibility of a future move but the team resolved to wait and see whether AB was of the same mind regarding a move following her discharge from the ward. Also at home AB was observed completing hot drinks safely and independently. Whilst in hospital she had also been able to complete her personal care independently so there were no concerns with her abilities.

On-going support and evaluation

AB was thought to benefit from regular compliance with anti-psychotic drug treatment alongside psychological and social support. She gradually improved and all involved in her care felt that they had contributed to this. She became more prepared to think about what would help her when she left hospital and was less suspicious and hostile. Alongside this she took her anti-hypertensive drugs and her anti-diabetic tablets regularly. Her blood pressure was well-controlled and her diabetes reasonably well-managed, despite the fact that she refused to stick to her recommended diet. These aspects of her care were to be handed back to primary care following discharge.

Both AB and her daughter agreed that she had improved, although there continued to be debate about what should be accepted as 'normal' for her when well and what would be the best support system to set in place on discharge. Her daughter was put in touch with carers' support services and offered ongoing support from the team. She was also involved in work with her mother on identifying early signs of relapse and planning how to take action should they emerge.

At one team meeting AB announced that she had decided which community nurse should follow her up after discharge home and that she had decided to go to a local resource centre. These decisions were respected: the social worker facilitated the resource centre day care placement and visits took place prior to discharge. This added a further dimension – that of liaison between the team and staff from the resource centre, who came along to a ward team meeting to meet AB and talk about future possibilities in that setting. The day centre offered a broad range of activities including arts-based and skills-based options. They explained that they would review how she felt about the placement at regular intervals at a meeting to which both she and her daughter would be invited, along with any other people involved in her treatment and care, and would liaise closely with the social worker and mental health team.

Following discharge AB was on enhanced CPA, with social services review organised through the resource centre (a joint health and social care service which has its own occupational therapy staff) and CPA review organised by her community nurse, who had a major role in her ongoing care in administering and monitoring her depot anti-psychotic treatment. Whilst at the resource centre AB engaged in reminiscence, computers and writing sessions. She appeared to work best on a one-to-one basis in that setting. She was offered the opportunity to attend community literacy support but declined without giving a reason.

HONOS 65+ is a tool that the team sometimes employs to look at outcomes, although it only gives a broad picture and is not ideal for that purpose. In this case it did indicate improvement in a number of areas.

Other actions

At times during her admission, AB had been hostile to different members of the team. It was important to share, discuss and reflect on this as a team: we incorporate reflective practice in our work (Gibbs 1988). It also emerged that she had targeted other patients in a hostile manner on occasions. This was addressed by her key nurse and the ward team offered appropriate support to the individuals involved. It was thought that she found the mixed ward setting (where people with dementia were cared for alongside people with 'functional' illness) difficult to adjust to, as her previous admissions had been to younger adult wards with a different clientele.

The possibility of a community treatment order was discussed during pre-discharge planning meetings but not pursued, as the team felt that good relationships had been established and compliance should first be tested out after discharge.

Case study 2: Mrs CD

CD is a 71-year-old married woman with no previous psychiatric contact who was referred to the older people's mental health service by her general practitioner (GP), who described her as 'confused'. The first contact with her was a home visit carried out by the old age psychiatrist accompanied by a psychiatric trainee. CD was not sure why her GP had referred her, but soon started to describe how she had been troubled for over two years by hearing voices which she believed were being piped into her home from the security system of a nearby shop. She also believed that they could somehow see her using the system. She explained that she had been to complain about it to the police but they had been unable to help. She felt that it must be part of a hate campaign aimed at her and other members of her family.

Apart from this she was physically fairly fit and did all her own house work and shopping. She didn't take any regular medication, just occasional painkillers for joint pains.

She lived in a small bungalow with her husband, who was disabled from a stroke. She had been caring for him without any help since the stroke about three years previously, which had left him with severely impaired mobility and difficulty in talking. It emerged during the assessment that he was in the bedroom nearby and the trainee went through to meet with him. CD and her husband had no children but she did have two older brothers living locally. Her mother had died of dementia but there was no other family history of contact with mental health services, and she herself had been a shop-worker until she retired at the age of 60. Since then her main interest had been running the home.

She described her sleep as disturbed by the things she was hearing, but was eating normally and had not lost weight. Her mood was quite cheerful despite the experiences she described. She thought at times that the shop staff were trying to hypnotise her and, on a few occasions, had thought that they were pumping some kind of gas into her bungalow. She also believed that they knew what she was thinking about as they often said out loud what she was thinking at the time. Her memory was tested using the Mini-mental State Examination (MMSE) (Folstein, Folstein and McHugh 1975) and she scored 29 out of 30, i.e. within the normal range.

Assessment approaches

This was CD's first contact with the mental health service and the phenomena described fitted with a diagnosis of schizophrenia. With a new illness it is important to check the person's memory in case they are developing organic brain disease, but there was no suggestion of any symptoms or signs of this in talking with CD and her husband, and her score on the MMSE was within the expected range. The other likely diagnosis for a new psychotic illness would be a depressive psychosis and this was considered, as she had sleep disturbance and the voices sometimes said threatening and upsetting things to CD. It was thought to be an unlikely explanation for her illness as her mood appeared bright to mental health staff and to her husband, and she had no other biological symptoms to suggest a major depression. In addition, her reaction to the psychotic experiences was not depressive, e.g. she went to complain to the police and described at times shouting back at the voices she heard and getting angry about their interference in her life.

Part of the assessment related to her role as carer to her husband and the team felt it was important to help her realise that she could be helped in caring for him as she was felt to be under a great deal of stress caring for him single-handed. This work involved mainly the occupational therapist and social worker, supported by the community psychiatric nurse. The occupational therapist looked at CD's home environment to see what practical changes would help with her husband's care and her own mental health and how activities/meaningful occupation might be of benefit. Safety was also considered. Initially a straightforward checklist was followed looking at mobility, transfers and all aspects of daily living. Leisure activities were also investigated, as it appeared that CD no longer pursued any interests as she spent all her time looking after her husband. She maintained that her GP had told her that nothing could be done to help with her husband's disabilities and that she would have to struggle on alone. Through the assessment several factors were noted from an occupational therapy perspective. Aspects of the environment were problematic, so equipment was prescribed to alleviate possible danger. This included the provision of grab rails, chair raisers, bathing and toilet equipment, mainly for use by her husband. The fire service was contacted to provide smoke alarms and a fire safety check. The potential role of assistive technology (Telecare) was also considered. This type of equipment can identify risks such as heat, floods and gas, can act as reminders for medication and can call for help if a person has fallen. A help centre or relative can be contacted automatically if any of the above problems occur in the home. This helps to maximise people's ability to live independently at home, prevents unnecessary hospital admissions and can reduce risk of injury. The provision of assistive technology may also be needed to enable a carer to continue the care of someone at home (Department of Health 2003).

This assessment linked with the social worker, who not only assessed CD's needs but carried out a carer's assessment with both partners, as the team recognised that both partners were caring for one another. Social networks were also considered and explored, in particular Mr and Mrs D's relationship with her older brothers. Mr D was referred to the physical and sensory team because of mobility problems. He was found to have some cognitive impairment following his stroke together with difficulties with activities of daily living.

Intervention

Negotiating a drug treatment plan with CD was a delicate matter as she had no insight. She agreed that she was stressed by her experiences and that seemed to offer common ground for considering how to help her. She agreed to see members of the CMHT for older people and to consider some medication to help with her mental health and her sleep. A sedative anti-psychotic was therefore prescribed and the community nurse subsequently followed her up. The risk benefit assessment relating to the anti-psychotic indicated that an atypical was preferable and that it should be introduced cautiously and under close community supervision. Since CD was sleep deprived and exhausted by caring, a sedative drug was thought to be indicated but this might improve her sleep at the expense of stopping her hearing when her husband needed her in the night (he was described as noisy at night-time).

In relation to CD's role as carer, as a first step she was sent some information on services for stroke that might support her and her husband in the community, and team members spent some time discussing with both partners what might help. It was felt that to some extent the way to CD's care was through her husband's care and the two were closely interlinked, needing an emphasis on collaboration and negotiation. Mr D's GP (unfortunately based at a separate practice from his wife's GP which complicated matters) was asked to review his medication as it was thought likely that his compliance was erratic. Both partners had their medication put into blister packs to simplify compliance. Mr D agreed to attend day care and this was arranged for two days each week in order to get him out of the house and to relieve some of the stress on his wife. Prior to this his wife had been locking him in the house while she did the shopping and then worrying all the time she was out that he might have fallen or come to some other harm. Now she was able to shop on the days he was at the day centre. Care link was also supplied. Her initial response was that she didn't want to consider having carers to help with Mr D, but this was kept open for future discussion. It emerged during the assessment that CD was not coping well with the couple's finances: in the past Mr D had done all of this, but had been unable to do so since his stroke. Appointeeship was raised as an issue and advance planning was also discussed, in particular whether a Lasting Power of Attorney might be applicable and helpful. One issue flagged for the future was the possibility of moving to a warden controlled extra-care setting where the couple would be able to have much more intensive support.

Mr D's attendance at day care opened up the possibility of his wife being able to benefit from participation in leisure activities. Taking part in leisure activities is known to be beneficial to physical well-being, social functioning, mental health and intellectual development and whilst leisure activities neither cure nor eradicate the effects of ageing or health difficulties, they introduce the potential to improve an individual's quality of life (Suto 1998, Ball *et al.* 2007). CD was given an information booklet to look at, listing all activities within the local area for people over the age of 50. It was felt that if she could make choices about leisure activities in which she had a particular interest, the occupational therapist could initially facilitate this with her at the times her husband was being cared for by someone else. It was further suggested that she might benefit by having the opportunity to participate in relaxation and anxiety management sessions as her stress was clearly a factor in her current difficulties. Weekly relaxation sessions were carried out with her in her home environment, and she attended a weekly anxiety management group run by occupational therapists in the community. Another area explored with CD was voluntary work. As she had been a former shop-worker it was thought that she might like to return to a similar environment in order to broaden her social focus within the community. The local Age Concern office was contacted and details given to CD about volunteering opportunities available locally. The local Stroke group was also contacted and agreed, with the couple's consent, to visit the couple to offer support and advice.

Both partners were regarded as vulnerable, and the team discussed safeguarding issues (although the formal safeguarding route was not pursued). Mr D was being locked in when his wife went to the shops, but day care was introduced along with Telecare interventions including door sensors and fall detectors.

At one stage the option of involving the older adult home treatment team was discussed as they would be able to co-ordinate and constantly evaluate treatment, but CD wanted to maintain control and opted not to go down this route. Instead the team agreed goals with her and regularly evaluated progress in weekly community team meetings alongside regular reviews with the couple in their home.

On-going support and evaluation

Evaluation of the interventions was mainly through observation and discussion. Prior to the programme of anxiety management sessions CD was asked to complete the Hospital Anxiety and Depression Scale (Zigmond and Snaith 1983). This was then repeated after the programme had ended. The scores showed a significant improvement when the programme had finished. Before and after each relaxation session CD was asked to rate herself on how anxious and tense she felt herself to be on a scale from feeling very anxious to feeling calm and relaxed. After almost every relaxation session she reported that she felt calmer and that the sessions had helped. When the anxiety management group had finished and CD appeared to be pursuing leisure activities independently she was discharged from the occupational therapy service, although because all team members attend the weekly community team meeting, everyone is kept up to date on people's progress in the community and can become re-involved quickly should the need arise.

For several months CD needed encouragement from team members to continue developing her hobbies and interests, in conjunction with day care for her husband and later the introduction of a sitting service. She gradually expressed fewer psychotic ideas, and settled into a routine (with support) which she reported to be less stressful and more enjoyable, although her husband's health continued to be a worry. Social services involvement now focused predominantly on her husband's care, which was regularly reviewed.

There were confidentiality issues with the neighbours as CD had been shouting at them in the street around the time of referral, and she worried that the neighbours would see team members visiting her and think she was mad. There was one neighbour who had been a friend some years before and as she improved she started to see this friend again and re-established her previous friendship. To some extent this alleviated her concerns about what people in the street might think.

Other actions

CD's case was discussed within clinical supervision in order to reflect on the intervention, evaluation and outcomes. It was agreed that her social network had been broadened through the interventions employed and her treatment overall was considered to be person-centred as all aspects of her life had been considered. It also fitted with the recovery model.

Voluntary organisations were involved through Age Concern and the sitting service was provided by Crossroads. Befriending was considered but proved not to be necessary as the other interventions had enabled CD to extend her social network.

A safeguarding case conference involving the vulnerable person's police officer was considered as an option but the safeguarding issues were addressed informally. The police were already aware of the couple as Mrs D had complained to them about her psychotic experiences on a number of occasions.

Discussion and conclusion

Working with people with a psychosis in later life can be rewarding and fulfilling for staff, although it brings a number of challenges which these two cases illustrate. There is a dearth of evidence about assessment and intervention for older adults with psychosis – most work has centred on younger people's services with emphasis on early intervention and the recovery model. These aspects of services have been less influential in older people's mental health. Working with people who lack insight into their psychosis necessitates careful negotiation of a therapeutic relationship. Communication can be complex. When a number of staff members are working with one family, co-ordination of interventions may involve a great deal of effort, liaison and trust between different team members. Team meetings are an important forum in maintaining communication and facilitating co-ordination. Psychological interventions for people with a psychosis are probably less well established in older people's mental health services, and this is an area needing service development. Self-help groups (e.g. the Hearing Voices Network) are also more commonly aimed at users of younger adult services and may not be as user-friendly or welcoming for older adults. The concept of 'recovery' is more often associated with younger adult services, although equally applicable and useful to older adults. Even a relatively simple matter such as choosing an anti-psychotic drug may be influenced by considerations of age, because of concerns about vascular risk with atypical anti-psychotics.

One of the problematic areas can be the differences in services between general psychiatry and older people's mental health, and the question of whether and when transfer is helpful for a person who is growing old with a psychotic illness. AB transferred in an emergency and this was not ideal. Sometimes older people's services are less well resourced and people may be disadvantaged by a service move, although the strong community emphasis in our service, where newly referred people are routinely assessed at home and follow-up appointments are normally carried out in the community, can be advantageous and may improve engagement with the mental health service in the longer term once the short-term disadvantage of disrupting established relationships has been overcome.

The most important aspects of working with both these families were felt to be threefold: ensuring communication between team members and with the families; partnership working between colleagues, agencies and between staff and family; and the ability to tailor care packages to the individuals and families concerned.

References

Age Concern and the Mental Health Foundation (2006) *Promoting mental health and well-being in later-life: A first report of the UK inquiry into mental health and well-being in later life*, London: Age Concern and the Mental Health Foundation. Available: www.mhilli.org (accessed 4 February 2010).

Almeida, O.P., Howard, R., Levy, R. and David, A.S. (1995a) 'Psychotic states arising in late life (late paraphrenia. The role of risk factors', *British Journal of Psychiatry*, 166: 215–28.

——(1995b) 'Psychotic states arising in late life (late paraphrenia) psychopathology and nosology', *British Journal of Psychiatry*, 166: 205–14.

Atwal, A., McIntyre, A., Craik, C. and Hunt, J. (2008) 'Occupational therapists' perceptions of predischarge home assessments with older adults in acute care', *British Journal of Occupational Therapy*, 71: 52–58.

Ball, V., Corr, S., Knight, J. and Lewis, M.J. (2007) 'An investigation into the leisure occupations of older adults', *British Journal of Occupational Therapy*, 70: 393–99.

Care Services Improvement Partnership (2007) *Age Equality: what does it mean for older people's mental health services? (Guidance Note)*, Available: www.olderpeoplesmentalhealth.csip.org.uk/everybodys-business/download-documents.html (accessed 4 February 2010).

Cohen, C.I., Magai, C., Yaffee, R. and Walcott-Brown, L. (2004) 'Racial differences in paranoid ideation and psychoses in an older urban population', *American Journal of Psychiatry*, 161: 864–71.

College of Occupational Therapists (2005) *College of Occupational Therapists Code of Ethics and Professional Conduct*, London: College of Occupational Therapists.

Creek, J. (2003) *Occupational therapy defined as a complex intervention*, London: College of Occupational Therapists.

Department of Health (1999) *National Service Framework for Mental Health*, London: Department of Health.

——(2001) *National Service Framework for Older People*, London: Department of Health.

——(2002) *Guidance on the single assessment process for older people*, Circular HSC 2002/001. Available: www.dh.gov.uk/en/SocialCare/Chargingandassessment/SingleAssessmentProcess/DH_079509#_5 (accessed 4 February 2010).

——(2003) *Guide to integrating community equipment services*, London: Department of Health.

——(2008) *Refocusing the care programme approach: Policy and positive practice guidance*. Available: www.dh.gov.uk/en/Publicationsandstatistics/Publications/PublicationsPolicyAndGuidance/DH_083647 (accessed 4 February 2010).

Department of Health and Care Services Improvement Partnership (2005) *Everybody's Business. Integrated Mental Health Services for Older Adults: A service development guide*, London: Care Services Improvement Partnership. Available: kc.csip.org.uk/upload/everybodysbusiness.pdf (accessed 4 February 2010).

Eyler Zorrilla, L.T. and Jeste, D.V. (2002) 'Late life psychotic disorders: nosology and classification', in J.R.M. Copeland, M.T. Abou-Saleh and G.G. Blazer (eds), *Principles and Practice of Geriatric Psychiatry*, 2nd edition, Chichester: John Wiley and Sons Ltd.

Faculty of Old Age Psychiatry (2006) *Raising the Standard: Specialist Services for Older People with Mental Illness*, Royal College of Psychiatrists. Available: www.rcpsych.ac.uk/PDF/RaisingtheStandardOAPwebsite.pdf (accessed 4 February 2010).

Folstein, M.F., Folstein, S. and McHugh, P. (1975) 'Mini-mental state: a practical method for grading the cognitive state of patients for the clinician', *Journal of Psychiatric Research*, 12: 189–98.

Gibbs, G. (1988) *Learning by doing. A guide to teaching and learning*, Oxford: Oxford Polytechnic.

Hong, C.S., Pearce, S. and Withers, R.A. (2000) 'Occupational therapy assessments: how client-centred can they be?', *British Journal of Occupational Therapy*, 63: 316–18.

Howard, R., Rabins, P.V., Seeman, M.V., Jeste, D.V. and the International Late-Onset Schizophrenia Group (2000) 'Late-onset schizophrenia and very-late-onset schizophrenia-like psychosis: an international consensus', *American Journal of Psychiatry*, 157: 172–78.

Howard, R.J., Graham, C., Sham, P., Dennehey, J., Castle, D.J., Levy, R. and Murray, R. (1997) 'A controlled family study of late-onset non-affective psychosis (late paraphrenia)', *British Journal of Psychiatry*, 170: 511–14.

Johnson, S. (1996) 'Activity Analysis', in A. Turner, M. Foster and S. Johnson (eds), *Occupational therapy and physical dysfunction: principles, skills and practice*, 4th edition, London: Churchill Livingstone.

Karim, S. and Byrne, E.J. (2005) 'Treatment of psychosis in elderly people', *Advances in Psychiatric Treatment*, 11: 286–96.

McCormack, B. (2004) 'Person-centredness in gerontological nursing: an overview of the literature', *International Journal of Older People Nursing* in association with the *Journal of Clinical Nursing*, 13 (3a): 31–38.

Ostling, S. and Skoog, I. (2002) 'Psychotic symptoms and paranoid ideation in a nondemented population-based sample of the very old', *Archives of General Psychiatry*, 59: 53–59.

Roper, N., Logan, W. and Tierney, A. (1981) *Learning to use the process of nursing*, Edinburgh: Churchill Livingstone.

Royal College of Psychiatrists (2004) *The Interface Between General and Community Psychiatry and Old Age Psychiatry Services: Report of a Working Group*, London: Royal College of Psychiatrists. Available: www.rcpsych.ac.uk/pdf/Interface.pdf (accessed 4 February 2010).

——(2009) *Links not boundaries: service transitions for people growing older with enduring or relapsing mental illness*, College Report 153, London: Royal College of Psychiatrists.

Sumsion, T. (2000) 'A revised occupational therapy definition of client-centred practice', *British Journal of Occupational Therapy*, 63 (7): 304–9.

Suto, M. (1998) 'Leisure in occupational therapy', *Canadian Journal of Occupational Therapy*, 65: 271–78.

World Health Organization (2007) *ICD*. Available: www.who.int/classifications/icd/en/bluebook.pdf (accessed 4 February 2010).

Zigmond, A.S. and Snaith, R.P. (1983) 'The Hospital Anxiety and Depression Scale', *Acta Psychiatrica Scandinavica*, 67: 361–70.

6 Alcohol and dual diagnosis in older people

Rahul (Tony) Rao, Rachael Buxey and Kadiatu (Kadia) Jalloh

Key messages

- Despite a growing prevalence of alcohol misuse in older people, there remains a dearth of service provision for alcohol misuse and dual diagnosis in older people.
- Socio-economic deprivation and ethnicity are strong risk factors for alcohol misuse in all age groups, but others such as social isolation and depression are common associations with hazardous and harmful drinking in later life.
- Although the general principles of assessment and treatment of alcohol misuse in older people are the same as for younger people, different methods of screening and management in the community are required.
- The implementation of new services requires both knowledge and skills, but also constantly re-evaluating their application to clinical practice in 'learning by doing' and sharing of specialist expertise.

Introduction

Terminology

Alcohol remains the nation's favourite drug. Drugs are chemicals that change the way that our bodies function, particularly our emotional state, behaviour and physical health. This may not always be associated with harm, but if an individual becomes addicted to drugs such as alcohol, certain changes will occur in the body that lead to symptoms of dependence. The 'classic' presentation is of a dependence syndrome (see below). However, older people may not fulfil all the criteria for dependence syndrome despite having serious problems related to the alcohol use or misuse.

Alcohol dependence syndrome

The World Health Organization (1993) states that a definite diagnosis of dependence should usually be made only if three or more of the following have been present together at some time during the previous year:

- Strong desire to drink alcohol.
- Difficulties in controlling alcohol intake (onset, termination, or levels of use).
- Physiological 'withdrawal state' when alcohol use ceases/reduces, with use of same (or closely related) substance to relieve or avoid these symptoms.

- Evidence of tolerance (increased dose of substance required to achieve effects originally produced by lower doses).
- Progressive neglect of alternative pleasures or interests owing to alcohol use, because of increased amount of time to obtain, take or recover from effects of alcohol.
- Persisting with alcohol use despite clear awareness of harm to physical/mental health.

In this chapter, the term 'older people' will refer to people of non-working age (65 and over). The main reason for this definition is that the difference between service provision for younger and older adults in the United Kingdom (UK) traditionally falls at this age cut-off point. In addition, the latter population has a very different profile in terms of health, social function and profiles of substance misuse, compared with people of working age.

Demographics and prevalence

Alcohol misuse is associated with considerable morbidity. In Europe, the disease burden attributable to alcohol (as measured by Disability Adjusted Life Years) represents the third most common risk factor, second only to high blood pressure and smoking.

About two-thirds of British men and one-third of women aged 65 and over, drink alcohol at least once a week; 19 percent of men and 5 percent of women in the same age group drink more than four and three units (termed 'sensible limits'), respectively, on any one day. There has been an increase in the percentage of older people exceeding recommended weekly drinking limits by about 60 percent in men and by over 100 percent in women between 1984 and 2006. Given that the UK population of over 65s is set to rise from 9 million to 12 million over the next 25 years, the public health implications of alcohol misuse in older people will continue to grow. This may be especially important for populations that are at particular risk, such as certain black and minority ethnic groups (e.g. older Irish people), particularly in areas of high socio-economic deprivation (Rao, Wolff and Marshall 2008).

Alcohol-related deaths and admissions to hospital have risen considerably over the past 15 years in the UK. In 1991–2006 alcohol-related mortality rose by nearly 90 percent in men in the 55–74 age group. In the UK, Scotland shows the highest prevalence of alcohol-related deaths, with over three times the number of age-standardised male deaths and over two times the number of female deaths compared with England, in the 55–74 age group. Although the north-west of England has the highest prevalence of such mortality in younger age groups, London has the highest prevalence in the over 75 age group. This is magnified in boroughs with high levels of deprivation. Given that the number of older people in the UK will increase by 50 percent between 2001 and 2031, there will continue to be a growing need to develop services to manage older people who misuse alcohol (Coulton 2009).

In addition to ethnicity, other factors influence alcohol misuse in older people, notably the effect of socio-economic deprivation. Other influences include bereavement, depression, social isolation, retirement and immobility. All these factors are more common in older than in younger people and may have considerable implications for the perpetuation of alcohol misuse in older people.

Local demographic picture

Among people aged 65 and above, London has the highest rate of alcohol-related hospitalised admissions in England, and Southwark (particularly in the north of the borough) has one of the highest rates of such admissions in London. Older people in Southwark therefore represent a population at high risk of alcohol misuse. Within the borough, there is as much as a five-fold difference in the rate of alcohol-related admissions between different electoral wards.

A prospective study of community team referrals to the North Southwark Older Adults Community Mental Health Services in 2002 found that of the people referred, 15 percent of those with alcohol dependence had depression. A cross-sectional study carried out a year later found that all 14 people on the team caseload, who reported drinking any alcohol at all, drank at hazardous or harmful levels.

Ethnicity has the greatest influence over alcohol misuse in Southwark, the borough in which the authors currently manage their clinical practice. Southwark has one of the highest populations of older Irish men in London and this population is known to have higher rates of alcohol misuse than the general UK population (Rao, Wolff and Marshall 2008). Ireland has the highest average yearly alcohol consumption and the highest prevalence of binge drinking in Europe (Ramstedt and Hope 2004). Coupled with the finding that older Irish people in Southwark have a higher prevalence of binge drinking and drinking above sensible limits compared with older people in Ireland (Rao, Wolff and Marshall 2008), the implications of these new findings have considerable relevance for the provision for alcohol services for older Irish people in Southwark.

Socio-economic factors are particularly relevant here, as Southwark is the third most deprived borough in London (Bardsley and Morgan 1996). Southwark represents a geographically unique borough in terms of alcohol misuse among older people. The catchment area of approximately 13,000 people aged 65 and over has a sizeable population with a history of heavy drinking, this being influenced by the large number of men who were previously employed on the docks and those with cultural influences on drinking behaviour, such as older Irish men traditionally employed in the construction industry. However, this 'culture' of drinking has also been incorporated into the lifestyle of a number of older women, irrespective of their previous occupation. As such, the provision of a home-based model of social care to improve independence and support older people with alcohol misuse remains a high priority. The Southwark service is 'fit for purpose' in that it mixes clinical expertise in a multi-disciplinary community mental health team to provide a seamless service in the detection, treatment and management of alcohol use disorders that is integrated within the borough's mental health of older people service. Such mental health expertise currently represents the only known sub-specialist service of this type in the UK and has arisen mostly through necessity, owing to the considerable burden of alcohol misuse in older people in North Southwark.

Policy considerations

There are a number of policy drivers for the care of people with alcohol misuse and dual diagnosis. It is unfortunate, however, that the vast majority of such policies make scant reference to the needs of older people.

The most recent policy having a direct bearing on services for alcohol misuse is the UK Government's *Alcohol Harm Reduction Strategy* (Cabinet Office, Prime Minister's Strategy Unit 2004). This document sets out four main objectives for reducing harm caused by alcohol, two of which have direct implications for the care of older people, namely attitudinal change from better education/communication and improving health/treatment services. A subsequent policy, entitled *Safe. Sensible. Social. The next steps in the National Alcohol Strategy* (Department of Health 2007), focused more heavily on the socio-economic costs of drinking in younger people, but outlined areas of general application such as a review of NHS alcohol spending, public information on 'sensible drinking' and local alcohol strategies. Indeed, the work carried out by the authors has informed the local alcohol strategy for Southwark, which is now incorporating good practice dual diagnosis service provision for older people. The *Cost of Alcohol Harm to the NHS in England* (Department of Health 2008) represents another key driver, which has provided evidence collated by the North West Public Health Observatory on the burden of alcohol-related illness and death already outlined above.

The *Dual Diagnosis Good Practice Guide* (Department of Health 2002a) suggests that mental health services take the lead for people with substance misuse and severe mental illness. Local Implementation Teams, in partnership with Drug and Alcohol Action Teams, are responsible for the implementation of the policy requirements described in the *Guide*. However, the potential benefit of age-specific dual diagnosis services is not highlighted. Although the rate of suicide in older men is higher than for any other age group, the Department of Health's *National Suicide Prevention Strategy for England* (Department of Health 2002b) again focuses on the clinical management of alcohol and drug misuse among young men who carry out deliberate self-harm.

Perhaps the most significant policy driver for the care of older people with alcohol misuse and dual diagnosis has been the *Supporting People Programme* (House of Commons 2004). This programme was set up to provide support services to vulnerable and older people, with the aim of delivering high quality and strategically planned housing-related services which are cost effective and reliable, and complement existing care services. The emphasis is on preventing tenancy breakdowns and promoting independence.

Other policies with potential influence are those that ensure adequate training and education for staff working with service users who misuse alcohol. The National Treatment Agency's *Drugs and Alcohol National Occupational Standards* (Skills for Health 2002) and the *Quality in Alcohol and Drug Services* organisational standards from Alcohol Concern and Standing Conference on Drug Abuse (1999) have both been instrumental in setting minimum standards for skills in meeting the objectives of service delivery. There has also been heightened awareness within the voluntary sector about the relevance of alcohol misuse in older people and the implications for services provided by a range of agencies (Age Concern and the Mental Health Foundation 2006).

In Southwark, a five-year strategy (2005–10) set out a number of key priorities for vulnerable adults and older people, one of which was specialist support to older people with mental health problems and alcohol misuse. The floating support service complements the care provided by the local mental health of older adults team and social services, with the main service outcome being the principle of social inclusion and recovery.

Applying principles

About our team

North Southwark Community Team for Older People is a multi-disciplinary community mental health team (CMHT) responsible for the assessment and treatment of older people with mental disorders, covering a large inner-city area of south-east London, UK. The CMHT comprises a Consultant Psychiatrist, Staff Grade doctor, four Community

Psychiatric Nurses (CPN), two Occupational Therapists, a Consultant Clinical Psychologist, an Assistant Psychologist and a Social Worker. The team is unique in offering a service based on what is now termed 'new ways of working' (Department of Health 2005), but was originally something of an anachronism, in that the service was set up in 1981, long before such a concept became recognised more widely.

The service (called the 'Guy's model') was the first 'open access' service for older people's mental health in the UK, accepting referrals from any source and offering a system of multi-disciplinary assessment and case management across the range of specialties. It remains one of the few services in the country that has doctors as care co-ordinators/key workers, thereby allowing a 'hands-on' approach to care and an in-depth experience of day-to-day management problems. This has been particularly advantageous in the area of alcohol misuse and dual diagnosis, where the Consultant Psychiatrist (RR) is care co-ordinator for older people who present with complex management problems relating to alcohol misuse, sharing expertise and seeking help from other specialities when required.

In response to the considerable number of referrals for older people with alcohol misuse who were unable to access more traditional substance misuse services, the team's consultant psychiatrist acquired expertise in the area of alcohol misuse, thereby enabling knowledge and skills to be shared with the rest of the CMHT. This has been helped by the creation of a specialised support service (Older Adults Support in Southwark – OASIS), which is jointly funded by *Supporting People* and Southwark Social Services. The benefit to older people with alcohol misuse and dual diagnosis has been demonstrated by a reduction in the number of older people admitted to hospital from North Southwark by over 90 percent over a five-year period. The impact of the CMHT and OASIS partnership led to North Southwark Community Team being awarded a Clinical Governance Award in the category of 'choice and empowerment' by South London and Maudsley NHS Foundation Trust in 2006.

The case study below marked a significant landmark in the development of the team's expertise in alcohol misuse and dual diagnosis, as it was following the assessment and treatment of this older person's addiction problem that the CMHT started to learn about how best to approach the management of alcohol misuse in older people. Prior to the management of Mr B, the service was ill-equipped in its knowledge and skills to manage similar service users. It was the ward/CMHT consultant who initially instigated the specialised ward assessment and referral to the CMHT; one that has resulted in Mr B remaining under the care of North Southwark Community Team three years later.

Case study

Mr B, a 68-year-old Caucasian man, was referred to the CMHT by his housing officer, following concerns about his mental state and vulnerability. Mr B had presented himself to her on several occasions over the previous six months, having mislaid the keys to his home. Mr B was also known to be living in a state of squalor.

At assessment, Mr B reported that he did not suffer from 'any kind of mental health problem', although he later admitted to 'feeling low'. A poignant statement by Mr B reflected the context of his drinking pattern, stating that 'I have nothing to do the entire day. I get bored and that is the reason why I drink'. In addition to feeling low in mood, Mr B complained of a low energy level, loss of interest in all previously enjoyable activities, low self-esteem and poor concentration. He also reported that he was eating poorly, had lost weight and that 'I cannot sleep for more than 15 minutes without getting up'. Passive suicidal ideas were reported in that he thought that he would be 'better off dead', but there were no active plans to end his own life.

There had been two previous admissions to mental health wards (one of these being under the *Mental Health Act* (1983)), but details were sketchy. Mr B had no known forensic history. There was a history of head injury after being mugged, but this did not lead to any long-lasting changes in cognitive function. Mr B was blind in one eye, owing to an injury several years before, but the sight in the remaining eye did not pose a significant social handicap. Mr B was not taking any prescribed or 'over the counter' medication on admission.

Background

Mr B was an only child who was born and schooled in London. He suffered a traumatic early childhood; his mother suffered physical abuse at the hands of his father, resulting in his parents separating when he was three years old. Between the ages of three and seven, Mr B lived with a relative in Scotland and then went to boarding school, reporting 'I hated every second of it'. However, he flourished at music, achieving a high level of ability in playing the trumpet. After leaving school with 'average grades' at the age of 16, he played the trumpet in various bands on a freelance basis. Mr B then joined a jazz band and released two records, but had not taken part in performing or playing the trumpet since the age of 50.

Mr B married at 30, but his wife later separated from him to live with one of his best friends, taking his son with her. This had a long-term impact on Mr B's self-esteem. In spite of having a few short-term relationships since then, there have been no enduring friendships or relationships and no friends or family in contact with him.

Mr B is an ex-smoker, quitting over 10 years previously. He has never used illicit substances or misused over the counter medication. He first drank alcohol in his teens, drinking socially at weekends. During his time gigging in bars and clubs, his alcohol use extended into evening drinking, during weekdays and then at lunchtimes. By the time Mr B was in his late 40s, he had changed from beer to spirits and escalated his alcohol consumption to at least half a bottle of vodka per day. This developed into a full dependence syndrome, resulting in his giving up his music career. He always drank in pubs and never at home, and drank steadily throughout the week. This has led to being mugged on a regular basis and to a neglect of all domestic activities of daily living such as cooking, cleaning and managing his finances. Mr B stated that he had not opened letters for several months, saying 'I have buried my head in the sand for a long time'. Over the two weeks prior to assessment, Mr B was drinking over 150 units of alcohol per week. Considering that the cut-off level for 'harmful drinking' is 50 units per week for men, Mr B was drinking considerably more than this level of misuse.

At first assessment, Mr B was dressed in unwashed clothes, smelling of urine, with an unshaven appearance and unwashed hair. There was no evidence of intoxication or alcohol withdrawal. He reported depressive symptoms as above, but there were no abnormal ideas of experiences suggestive of a psychotic disorder. On cognitive testing, there was no evidence of cognitive impairment. Mr B had partial insight into his problems, agreeing to engage with any help that was thought necessary, but showed no awareness of his depression or alcohol misuse. He was admitted to an acute psychiatry ward for older people. Blood investigations and physical examination showed no obvious evidence of alcohol-related physical harm. A dual diagnosis of alcohol dependence syndrome accompanied by moderate depressive disorder was made.

General assessment

Mr B was assessed at initial referral with a standardised, locally developed generic assessment tool for use by clinicians from different health backgrounds. The assessment interview incorporates several prompts in each of the areas relevant to a full mental health assessment and has undergone a number of revisions over the years, having been first piloted by North Southwark Community Team for Older People. The assessment tool has been supplemented by questions covering alcohol use, particularly estimations of quantity/ frequency of alcohol consumption. Following hospital admission, the consultant (who was also the community responsible medical officer) was able to implement a more specialised assessment that covered substance misuse history and associated physical and mental health problems. This was able to identify pre-disposing (e.g. genetic and early life experiences), precipitating and maintaining factors for his alcohol misuse and enabled a diagnosis of both alcohol dependence syndrome and depressive disorder. This approach is set out below, in further detail.

Mr B spent six months on the in-patient ward, during which time considerable progress was made in addressing his alcohol misuse and treating his depression. In fact, the admission also served to highlight behaviours and attitudes that had become ingrained and maladaptive, shedding light on Mr B's inability to function independently in the community. For example, he preferred to eat in his room and left his room in an untidy state, often hoarding food underneath his bed. Although the hospital admission was protracted, owing to the considerable time required to clear and refurbish his flat, it allowed both in-patient and CMHT professionals to engage with Mr B and to implement interventions over a long period of time before final discharge in summer 2006. This discharge was not without its set-backs, being punctuated by episodes of intoxication following extended periods of home leave.

Specialised assessment approaches in managing Mr B

History and examination

- Detailed alcohol misuse history.
  Includes age when first used substance(s) and evolution of substance use/misuse and associated factors, including quantity/frequency of use, number of units per week, harmful/hazardous level of use, presence/absence of dependence syndrome and use/misuse of other licit (e.g. nicotine/over the counter medication)/illicit (e.g. cannabis) substances.

- Alcohol assessment screening tools.
  These need to be age-specific, as many of the more traditional rating scales lack validity (e.g. they do not measure what they are supposed to be measuring). The Short MAST-G (Blow, Gillespie and Barry 1998) is commonly used, but others such as the Drinking Problems Index (Finney, Moos and Brennan 1991) and Alcohol-Related Problems Survey (Fink *et. al.* 2002) are used in more specialised settings.

- Psychosocial complications of alcohol misuse.
  These include family history of alcohol misuse, occupational risks (e.g. high-risk occupations such as working in construction industry/brewery), domestic violence and relationship problems, work record (e.g. lateness, sickness, dismissal for intoxication), forensic history (e.g. drink driving, public order offences), mental disorders (e.g. personality disorder, depression, cognitive impairment such as dementia), self-neglect, financial problems (e.g. rent arrears), decline in domestic activities, financial/social/sexual exploitation.

- Physical complications of alcohol misuse.
  These are numerous, but commonly affect stomach (ulceration), liver (alcoholic hepatitis, progressing to cirrhosis), blood (anaemia) and nervous system (peripheral neuropathy – lack of sensation in legs) and instability/falls related to episodes of intoxication. Falls may lead to head injury and the possibility of bleeding beneath the skull. Alcohol may also alter the way in which medication is metabolised by the body and can also add to the side-effects of drugs such as opiates (commonly found in prescribed painkillers).

Specialised investigations

- Neuro-imaging and Neuropsychological testing.
  Both of these investigations give a more precise idea of the nature (area of the brain affected) and severity of any damage to the brain associated with alcohol misuse. In younger people, the clinical picture of cognitive impairment is usually one of Korsakoff's Syndrome, which is confined to memory problems and is irreversible, as it involves bleeding into certain areas of the brain. However, the toxic effects of alcohol on the brain may become widespread in later life and become associated with dementia. Rather than irreversible changes attributable to bleeding, the brain may become damaged through loss of nerve terminals, and widespread changes in cognitive function then lead to dementia. There is evidence to suggest that this type of alcohol-related brain damage may recover to some extent, following abstinence from alcohol. This has significant consequences for encouraging abstinence in older people drinking at harmful levels.

- Nursing and medical observations.
  Nursing and medical observations are crucial in the assessment and monitoring of alcohol withdrawal, which ranges from symptoms that cause mild discomfort, through to a condition known as delirium tremens. The latter condition carries a 10 percent–15 percent risk of death if not treated promptly (Kraemer, Mayo-Smith and Calkins 1997). This is because delirium tremens has a major impact on the body, particularly in those people who already have other physical problems such as poor nutrition, dehydration and heart disease. The clinical assessment of alcohol withdrawal relies on medical expertise, but screening of classical withdrawal symptoms (e.g. tremor, sweating, agitation and sensory disturbance) can be undertaken by nursing staff.

Specialised interventions for Mr B

Mr B's engagement in the therapeutic process was essential prior to implementation of any intervention. It was first necessary to establish his motivation to change, using a

Stages of Change model (Prochaska and DiClemente 1992), which allowed a greater understanding of his motivation to change his drinking behaviour. In Mr B's case, he was in the 'pre-contemplation' phase of the cycle, in that he showed no immediate desire to change his drinking pattern. This reflected the purpose that alcohol served in his life: it helped him avoid issues and retreat into a 'safe place' where he did not have to take responsibility for his life. This maladaptive equilibrium was further perpetuated by the lack of social support and accompanying depression. Over the course of Mr B's initial hospital admission, depressive symptoms began to resolve and it then became possible to initiate a therapeutic relationship. However, a lack of self-esteem was a significant barrier to progress, with Mr B often telling the nursing staff that what he told the consultant in the ward round was 'what he (the consultant) wanted to hear'. This was addressed and reflected back to Mr B in the setting of motivational interviewing, which will be discussed later in the chapter.

Medical interventions (RR)

The immediate management of Mr B as an in-patient was to minimise the effects of alcohol withdrawal. This involved the initiation and tapering down of medication over a 10-day period, which reduced the severity of alcohol withdrawal symptoms. Once this was complete, it was necessary to supplement the body's depleted vitamin store with Vitamin B compound. Fortunately, there were no other physical complications requiring treatment. In addition to vitamin supplements, antidepressant treatment was also initiated, ensuring that the antidepressant was one that had fewer interactions with alcohol.

Psychological ward-based interventions (RR and RB)

After screening Mr B for his severity of alcohol misuse using the Short MAST-G, a Brief Intervention was carried out. Brief Interventions are two-fold in nature:

Stage 1: Brief Advice is given regarding sensible drinking and the harms associated with alcohol.

Stage 2: Motivational Enhancement Treatment is delivered, which is a systematic intervention approach using strategies derived from the principles of motivational psychology to enhance a person's own resources for changing the pattern of substance use (Saunders, Wilkinson and Phillips 1995).

It is known that Screening and Brief Intervention over a 25-minute session, followed by follow-up sessions, together are effective in the reduction of alcohol-related harm in older people (US Preventive Services Taskforce 2004). This approach was continued by the Consultant Clinical Psychologist upon discharge into the community, using a motivational interviewing approach.

Motivational interviewing is a psychological intervention, designed to help people identify and acknowledge their substance misuse and move towards cessation. It involves a non-confrontational approach that avoids labelling and accepts the perspective of the patient as a starting point from which to approach change. Using this 'Stages of Change' framework, ambivalence and relapse are acknowledged and viewed as opportunities to move the patient toward healthy outcomes. Specific events are used to shift the patient's perceptions about the consequences of the behaviour and to acquire insights into alternatives. A useful acronym for the techniques used in this treatment is FRAMES, which refers to the use of Feedback, Responsibility for change lying with the individual, Advice-giving, providing a Menu of change options, an Empathic counselling style, and the enhancement of Self-efficacy. The model is designed to be fluid and patients may often move between different stages at different times during treatment.

Two months prior to discharge, Mr B was assessed by RB (Consultant Clinical Psychologist). Mr B started by saying that he didn't know that he had been referred to Psychology and said he didn't really know what Psychology was. He maintained that he was in hospital because his flat was untidy and that he had not had any problems at home leading up to his admission, stating only that 'you have to work with the cards you have been dealt in life'. After some further discussion, he was able to acknowledge that at times he did feel a sense of personal loss in that he had not achieved more in his life. He said that he felt he had a lot of unrealised potential that seemed unreachable and impossible to activate, 'as if it was on just the other side of a misted-up window', but rapidly changing the subject with, 'I'm doing alright really'.

Although denying the depression with which he had been diagnosed, Mr B reported that he been admitted to hospital to stop drinking and that was 'a good thing' because he had been drinking one-to-two bottles of vodka a day. This, he said, 'gets me up to go out and do something'. He also said that he felt no ill effects from the amount of alcohol he was drinking and had never had a hangover and never 'got drunk', and later mentioning that drinking was bad for his health and that he did not want to 'end up on a dialysis machine'. Mr B was very reluctant to talk about his personal life, only stating that his wife had left him for his best friend 40 years ago and that his last long-term relationship had ended in 1990, that it had been a very difficult time for him as well, and that he hadn't felt like starting another intimate relationship with anyone since then. When asked to keep a diary of his thoughts and feelings, he said 'a chap like [him] doesn't have thoughts and feelings' and 'that's the sort of thing you learn when you go to university'.

On-going support and evaluation

Clinical psychology (RB)

Working psychologically with Mr B has been an unusual and rewarding experience. When I first met him, I thought it unlikely that he would engage with psychology services because he seemed to have very little insight and to think very concretely about most things. However, I have now been working with him for nearly three years and he has made a lot of progress over that time. I think it is often the human and humane aspects of our service which reach out to some of the 'difficult to reach/engage' people who are referred, and enables them to stay in contact and engage with the service. With Mr B, notable examples of this include:

- Home visits.
- Accompanying him to court on several occasions.
- Accompanying him to visits to local amenities including libraries, day centres and the general practitioner (GP) surgery.
- Helping him communicate with and advocating for him in negotiations with banks, debt agencies and services like gas, water and electricity.

However, these aspects would not be helpful without being embedded within the community multidisciplinary team service which has experience of, and knowledge about, working with older people with mental health and substance misuse issues.

Mr B continues to express himself in a very concrete way and often tells me he does not have thoughts or feelings. When I explore this further with him and demonstrate to him from the things he says to me that he *is* thinking and feeling, he laughs and as if for the sake of politeness will agree with me that, 'Well, I suppose I must do then'.

He told me when I first met him, and repeats this still, that he was taken into hospital because his flat was untidy, and mostly he still holds this view. He can only agree that he has changed and made progress if prompted to and given concrete examples (e.g. attending college courses, picking up the trumpet again and getting a band together – which has now had several public performances). He does not like 'complainers' and will never complain himself, consistently refusing to complete psychological evaluation forms because he sees it as 'complaining'. However, when he seemed very low a few months ago, I persuaded him for the first time to fill in a Beck Depression Inventory (Beck, Steer and Brown 1996), in which he scored 35 in the severe range and then did not want to talk about any of his answers that were of concern to me. Despite these challenges we have established a therapeutic rapport and continue to work together on his general feeling of being low in energy and motivation and on his ongoing sense of *ennui*.

Medical review (RR)

The first year after discharge from hospital was a time of immense turmoil in Mr B's life, particularly given the dissonance between the life that he had previously led and the input that he started to receive from the CMHT. My main role as Mr B's Consultant Old Age Psychiatrist was to undertake regular reviews of his mental state and risk (particularly suicide risk), as well as overseeing the general direction of progress.

Using a non-judgemental, motivational interviewing model combined with Mr B's own cognitive resources to address difficulties, a period of stability was achieved, during which he remained compliant with antidepressant medication and experienced periods of abstinence lasting for weeks at a time. These were interspersed with episodes of binge drinking, which were 'reframed' during my reviews as temporary setbacks rather than a 'failure to maintain abstinence'. It was noticeable that there were certain triggers to a relapse in alcohol misuse, particularly financial concerns and moving flat. During episodes of heavy drinking, Mr B would cut himself off completely from services for days at a time, but our approach was always to give him space and choice over how he engaged with us, whilst at the same time monitoring risk carefully. However, as mentioned above, there was often a disparity between Mr B's impression of his life and what he actually did (for example college courses and playing in a band).

Older adults support service in Southwark-OASIS (EK – see acknowledgements)

OASIS came into existence in April 2005, being a joint venture by the Older Persons Partnership Board and Health and Social Care Commissioners. It was recognised that mainstream home care services often were not in a position to deliver the right level of services to older people with high level of need, particularly in the areas of alcohol misuse and self-neglect.

The role of OASIS was central to maintaining stability in Mr B's life, with harm minimisation, support, social inclusion and recovery being core features of engaging with him. Key to successful rehabilitation and recovery was the principle of 'doing with' rather than 'doing for'. Although there were some elements of the latter (e.g. clearing rubbish from flat), much of the activity scheduling also required Mr B's own input. He frequently complained of being 'bored with it all', but began to take part in a number of activities such as French lessons and music classes, taking up the trumpet for the first time in many years.

Supporting Mr B through change has also been essential. During OASIS involvement with Mr B, he has often cut himself off from services when drinking heavily, largely through his embarrassment at being seen intoxicated and being involved in fights. Similarly, moving flat and adjusting to new surroundings has been associated with similar situations. Throughout OASIS contact, Mr B has been given choices and opportunities to change his lifestyle, which he has started to do only after three years of contact.

Community Psychiatric Nurse input (KJ)

Since his discharge from hospital, Mr B has been managed by a care co-ordinator. Engaging Mr B has been challenging, largely because he discloses little about his thoughts and feelings, for fear of being judged in a negative light and because he does not like to complain. During periods of abstinence, positive affirmations have been productive, although the ongoing social isolation and lack of self-confidence make him vulnerable to deterioration in his mood. He has often used alcohol as a way of coping with boredom and loneliness, as well as 'blocking out' the stresses of everyday life when there is a period of change. Although Mr B often has only partial insight into the need for support and review, he has consistently adhered to taking antidepressant medication regularly, noting that his mood deteriorates within a week of the few attempts he has made to stop this. This insight has been evident from Mr B's comments about the link between his mood and taking antidepressant medication.

Multi-disciplinary approach to management

Although Mr B remains at significant risk of depression, social isolation and a relapse to alcohol dependence if not receiving the level of support that he still gets, the success in maintaining Mr B independently in the community for the past three years has relied on a consistent and co-ordinated approach from a number of health professionals and support staff. Clear lines of communication were required between CPN/OASIS staff and the Consultant Psychiatrist, particularly during periods of disengagement and over medico-legal matters. An electronic record of interventions also aided the communication process. Decision-making at the weekly multi-disciplinary meetings involved expertise from all those involved in Mr B's care, as well as frequent reviews and changes to risk management. The fact that there had been no attempts at self-harm and a progressive improvement in health and social functioning, bears witness to the range and depth of interventions employed and the management of risk on a day-to-day basis. The recovery model used has also resulted in recognition from the Mental Health Trust of excellence in service delivery and it is because of the success in managing Mr B by combining knowledge and skills within the CMHT that the framework of management has been applied to other older people with alcohol misuse on the team caseload. The model has also been recognised as one of good practice both locally and nationally.

Discussion and conclusion

Good practice is not just about modelling care on policies and procedures, but also about applying these to clinical care in a flexible and pragmatic way. This involves learning from experience, drawing upon outcomes and constantly re-shaping service delivery through discussion and skill sharing, in conjunction with listening carefully to the service user's viewpoint. For us, setting up a much needed service within existing resources was challenging, largely because we had nothing against which to compare ourselves, yet, at the same time, appreciating the need to innovate and implement good practice. Mr B is, and always was, a private man who would not engage with traditional services such as Alcoholics Anonymous, with treatment at a drop-in centre that would require self-referral. A home-based model of care was therefore the only way forward.

The first lesson learned from the case study above was that objective evidence of alcohol misuse in older people requires a careful and considered approach, with the possibility of resistance and disengagement creeping in and posing the risk of a complete loss of the therapeutic relationship. In Mr B's case it was also only possible to gauge the true severity of his alcohol misuse by using age-specific screening tools such as the Short MAST-G and indirect evidence of observed intoxication and self-neglect whilst in the community.

Unlike younger people with alcohol misuse, it was always important to consider the specific risk factors associated with Mr B's drinking. Although there were already predisposing factors such as a past history of alcohol misuse and possible untreated past episodes of depression, the interplay between personality attributes (particularly low self-esteem) and other more age-specific risk factors made his care planning and the delivery of interventions more challenging. Regarding the former risk factors, engaging Mr B when he was clearly depressed was problematic; even when this depression was ameliorated, his poor self-image and feeling of 'not deserving' services and 'not complaining' made resistance to change all the more prominent. Regarding age-specific risk factors, social isolation and resulting lack of close confidantes were recurrent triggers to relapse. Although an intelligent and articulate man, his talents with music and creativity were never fully realised; he saw himself as an 'alcoholic', as this was the way that others viewed him. Experience with both Mr B and other service users with alcohol misuse and dual diagnosis suggests social isolation to be a recurring theme in the perpetuation of alcohol misuse and is in keeping with the literature in this area (Hanson 1994).

The combination of approaches offered by the multi-disciplinary team also provided a constant shift of focus, with different clinicians intervening in different ways at different times. For example, when it was clear that Mr B's mood was deteriorating, the consultant (RR) had comparatively more contact, in order to monitor mood and suicide risk, as well as carrying out brief interventions and offering continuity of care between CMHT, ward and then CMHT again. There were times when the physical effects of alcohol misuse were more noticeable, which meant closer liaison with Mr B's GP. One poignant example was when Mr B complained of abdominal pain. By liaising with the GP, the prescription of a stomach acid lowering drug brought immense relief and might otherwise have gone undiagnosed.

Psychological interventions from the team Consultant Psychologist (RB) combined formal therapy such as supportive psychotherapy, cognitive behavioural therapy and motivational interviewing with practical help such as engaging with local resources. This support even extended to accompanying Mr B to court and making positive recommendations on his behalf.

Day-to-day social support from the OASIS team (EK) taught us valuable lessons in choice and empowerment. Although episodes of disengagement during periods of heavy drinking that could last for days initially concerned us, we began to realise that these were often short-term responses to crises such as financial problems or problems with self-esteem. Mr B clearly had a choice to drink, which was a downside of the abstinence-based model that he had chosen to follow. After bouts of drinking, when contact was resumed, he still valued the support from our CMHT, so these periods were viewed in a long-term context, with recognition of general progression in his recovery. The OASIS service was also a central driver for social engagement, working within both a harm reduction and social inclusion model. Encouraging Mr B to enrol in a local college and take up previously enjoyed musical activities had a two-fold benefit. The very fact that he was out of his flat and able to feel part of his local community and, indeed, mainstream society, meant that his exposure to alcohol was minimised and that his self-confidence could improve. At times, he resented the intensity of support and it became necessary to take a step back, sometimes observing risk from a distance. After all, Mr B had always found it difficult to form close therapeutic relationships and had not experienced the type of help in the past that he was presently receiving. In fact, Mr B later commented, 'they showed me that I was ill when I didn't realise that I was. I still get good days and bad days for no reason but I'm beginning to feel a bit more able to deal with it.'

The provision of a specific service to meet the needs of older people with alcohol misuse and dual diagnosis took 10 years to establish. The main obstacle was the need for this to be delivered within existing resources. In 1999 it was noted that between 10 percent and 20 percent of referrals to the CMHT per month involved alcohol misuse. By 2002 it was noted that up to 50 percent of in-patient admissions involved a dual diagnosis, with alcohol misuse being central to the clinical problems. The ward consultant (RR) recalls seeing older people admitted with alcohol-related dementia and thinking 'if only these people had been detected in the community at an early stage'.

In 2003 an audit of the community team caseload revealed that only 5 percent of the CMHT caseload showed evidence of alcohol misuse, but all those who did so were drinking at harmful limits. As a result, RR embarked on an MSc in clinical and public health aspects of additions, which enabled him to provide much-needed expertise in managing older people with substance misuse.

Five years on, following a series of awareness seminars to GPs in the catchment area and the provision of OASIS in 2005, the CMHT is finally able to manage alcohol misuse and dual diagnosis in older people more effectively. This has cut down the percentage of mental health admissions to less than 5 percent, with a doubling in the proportion of older people with dual diagnosis on the team caseload to 10 percent.

The CMHT now has a higher awareness and lower threshold for the detection of alcohol misuse and dual diagnosis, and so links service users to the necessary mental health expertise and social support, as well as with other statutory and voluntary agencies such as Southwark Irish Pensioners Project. Our CMHT nurses also now have access to training courses for the management of substance misuse within our Mental Health Trust, and RR has shared his knowledge and skills with the rest of the team, allowing empowerment of clinicians in service delivery. The acquisition of 'cultural competence' in the engagement of particular minority ethnic groups (especially the Irish population) has been an added benefit.

The journey began with Mr B, but has now extended to others with equally complex management problems. We continue to learn, evaluate, implement and modify treatment interventions. This has not been possible without access to a constantly changing knowledge base, most of which traditionally comes from the United States. However, given our success in this area, there is scope for spreading our good practice within the UK. Sharing our experiences with local resources such as the London Drug and Alcohol Network, and informing government policy have taken us a step closer to this objective, with our work actively informing the *All Party Parliamentary Group on Alcohol Misuse* (Alcohol Concern 2009).

Acknowledgements

The authors would like to thank Eva Kisitu (EK) for her role in managing the OASIS service and overseeing the service in its contribution to the care of older people with alcohol misuse in Southwark. Also, members of the Mental Health of Older Adults Service for their support and encouragement, as well as Southwark Irish Pensioners Project, Faculty of Addictions at the Institute of Psychiatry and the Trust's Dual Diagnosis groups.

References

Age Concern and the Mental Health Foundation (2006) *Promoting mental health and well-being in later-life: A first report of the UK inquiry into mental health and well-being in later life*, London: Age Concern and the Mental Health Foundation. Available: www.mhilli.org (accessed 4 February 2010).

Alcohol Concern (2009) *All Party Parliamentary Group on Alcohol Misuse: the future of alcohol treatment services*, London: Alcohol Concern.

Alcohol Concern and Standing Conference on Drug Abuse (1999) *QuADS: organisational standards for alcohol and drug treatment services*, London: Standing Conference on Drug Abuse.

Bardsley, M. and Morgan, D. (1996) *Deprivation and health in London*, London: Health of Londoners Project.

Beck, A.T., Steer, R.A. and Brown, G.K (1996) *Manual for Beck Depression Inventory II (BDI-II)*, San Antonio, TX: Psychology Corporation.

Blow, F.C., Gillespie, B.W. and Barry, K.L. (1998) 'Brief screening for alcohol problems in elderly populations using the Short Michigan Alcoholism Screening Test-Geriatric Version (SMAST-G)', *Alcoholism: Clinical and Experimental Research*, 22(Suppl.): 131A.

Cabinet Office, Prime Minister's Strategy Unit (2004) *Alcohol harm reduction strategy for England*, London: Cabinet Office.

Coulton, S. (2009) 'Alcohol use disorders in older people', *Reviews in Clinical Gerontology*, 19: 217–25.

Department of Health (2002a) *Dual Diagnosis Good Practice Guide*, London: Department of Health.

——(2002b) *National Suicide Prevention Strategy for England*, London: HM Government.

——(2005) *New ways of working for psychiatrists: Enhancing effective, person-centred services through new ways of working in multidisciplinary and multiagency contexts*, London: HM Government.

——(2007) *Safe. Sensible. Social. The next steps in the National Alcohol Strategy*, London: HM Government.

——(2008) *The Cost of Alcohol Harm to the NHS in England: An update to the Cabinet Office (2003) study*, London: HM Government.

Fink, A., Morton, S.C., Beck, J.C., Hays, R.D., Spritzer, K., Oishi, S. and Moore, A. (2002) 'The Alcohol-Related Problems Survey: Identifying hazardous and harmful drinking in older primary care patients', *Journal of the American Geriatrics Society*, 50: 1717–22.

Finney, J.W., Moos, R.H. and Brennan, P.L. (1991) 'The Drinking Problems Index: A measure to assess alcohol-related problems among older adults', *Journal of Substance Abuse*, 3: 395–404.

Hanson, B.S. (1994) 'Social network, social support and heavy drinking in elderly men – a population study of men born in 1914, Malmö, Sweden', *Addiction*, 89: 725–32.

House of Commons (2004) *Supporting Vulnerable and Older People: The Supporting People Programme*, Tenth Report of Session 2003–4, London: The Stationery Office.

Kraemer, K.L., Mayo-Smith, M.F. and Calkins, D.R. (1997) 'Impact of age on the severity, course and complications of alcohol withdrawal', *Archives of Internal Medicine*, 157: 2234–41.

Prochaska, J.O. and DiClemente, C.C. (1992) *Stages of Change in the Modification of Problem Behaviors*, Newbury Park, California: Sage.

Ramstedt, M. and Hope, A. (2004) 'Irish drinking habits of 2002 – Drinking and drinking-related harm in a European comparative perspective', in Health Promotion Unit, Department of Health and Children, *Strategic Task Force on Alcohol, Second Report*, Dublin.

Rao, R., Wolff, K. and Marshall. E.J. (2008) 'Alcohol use and misuse in older people: a local prevalence study comparing English and Irish inner-city residents living in the UK', *Journal of Substance Use*, 13: 17–26.

Saunders, B., Wilkinson, C. and Phillips, M. (1995) 'The impact of a brief motivational intervention with opiate users attending a methadone programme', *Addiction*, 90: 415–24.

Skills for Health (2002) *Drugs and Alcohol National Occupational Standards (DANOS)*, London: Skills for Health.

US Preventative Services Taskforce (2004) 'Screening and behavioral counselling interventions in primary care to reduce alcohol misuse: recommendation statement, *Annals of Internal Medicine*, 140: 554–56.

World Health Organization (1993) *International Classification of Diseases*, 10th edition, Geneva: World Health Organization.

7 Memory services

Psychological distress, co-morbidity and the need for flexible working – the reality of later life mental health care

Sue Watts, Lee Harkness, Rachel Domone, Gyll Shields, Gillian Moss and Nora Bilsborough

Key messages

- Drawing distinctions between older people with dementia and those with 'functional' non-organic mental health conditions is often difficult and sometimes impossible in practice.
- 'Off the shelf' therapies and packages of care may not be appropriate – treatment options must take account of the person's history and relationships together with current co-morbid mental and physical health.
- If older people do not respond to offered treatment, the fault may be in the service model, the practitioner's approach or level of specialist skill.
- Stigmatisation of older people and of dementia is a major obstacle affecting development and uptake of services.

Introduction

Epidemiology

It is estimated that the population of older people in the United Kingdom (UK) will grow from 9.6 million in 2005 to 12.7 million in 2021, with rates of dementia and other mental health problems increasing proportionately (Age Concern and the Mental Health Foundation 2006, 2007, Alzheimer's Society 2007). Over the next 15 years the number of older people with some form of mental health problem is predicted to increase to one in every 15 people. Research into the incidence and prevalence of dementia and other mental health problems shows considerable variation in rates due to different methodologies and measuring instruments utilised. However, a UK Inquiry suggests that approximately 5 percent of older people in the community are likely to have dementia; rising to between 50 percent and 80 percent of those in care homes (Age Concern and the Mental Health Foundation 2006, 2007). The *National Dementia Strategy* (Department of Health 2009a) estimates that approximately 700,000 people have dementia in the UK, of whom 570,000 live in England. In addition, 10 percent–15 percent of older people in the community are likely to have depression, rising to 40 percent in care homes. Both conditions may co-exist.

Until relatively recent times, management of dementia has been heavily influenced by negative stereotypes and an assumption that the person with dementia should be protected from knowledge of their own condition and its implications. However, over the last two decades, new pharmacological and psychosocial approaches to treatment have prompted a move toward therapeutic optimism and recognition of the value of early detection and disclosure of the diagnosis of dementia (Pratt and Wilkinson 2001). Wright and Lindesay (1995) charted the early development of memory clinics in the UK. Initially, many were hospital-based assessment and advice services linked to research projects. They were, however, 'ill-equipped to provide for the ongoing care needs of their patients and most rely on referral to the local health and social services for this' (Wright and Lindesay 1995: 383).

The licensing of new drugs to alleviate some of the symptoms of Alzheimer's disease had a significant impact on the further development of memory clinics. Donepezil (Aricept) was launched in 1997, Rivastigmine (Exelon) received its licence in 1998 and Galantamine (Reminyl) in 2000; see also the National Institute for Health and Clinical Excellence (NICE) Technology Appraisals (National Institute for Health and Clinical Excellence 2001, 2007) for the evidence base. In many instances clinics were set up specifically to ensure delivery of treatment with acetylcholinesterase inhibitors (AChEIs). Lindesay *et al.* (2002) found the number of memory clinics in the UK had doubled by 2000 and that they operated a broader range of service models.

During this period there has also been increasing evidence of effective outcomes from psychosocial interventions for early stages of dementia, e.g. Clare (2003) and Moniz-Cook *et al.* (2009). These interventions address ways of sharing the diagnosis of dementia, cognitive rehabilitation and stimulation techniques (Clare and Woods 2004, Alzheimer's Society 2007), and memory groups utilising varied therapeutic strategies (Cheston, Jones and Gilliard 2003), as well as more long-established interventions with carers (Charlesworth *et al.* 2008). This literature is not reviewed in detail here, but Moniz-Cook and Manthorpe (2009) have edited a wide-ranging, informative and accessible book covering the work of researchers and clinicians in the development and delivery of evidence-based clinical practice in psychosocial interventions for dementia. In this they also draw attention to the importance of tailoring psychosocial interventions for people with dementia to each individual's circumstances and preferences.

Developments arising from research were followed in 2001 by Standard Seven: Mental Health of the *National Service Framework for Older People* (Department of Health 2001), which emphasized the importance of achieving early diagnosis for older people with suspected dementia. The combined impacts of the *National Service Framework for Older People*, NICE Technology Appraisals (National Institute for Health and Clinical Excellence 2001, 2007) and the *National Dementia Strategy* (Department of Health 2009a) have seen a widespread increase in services. A majority of later life services now offer memory clinics which focus on diagnosis, provision of medication, education and support with adjustment to diagnosis. However, the availability of psychosocial interventions is much more variable.

Services are now sufficiently widespread that examples of good practice are recognised and have been evaluated (e.g. Croydon Memory Service: Bannerjee *et al.* 2007 [and see Chapter 8 of this book]; Hull Memory Clinic: Moniz-Cook *et al.* 2009). Clinical governance issues (Phipps and O'Brien 2002) and quality standards are also being addressed. An accreditation process has evolved from the North West Memory Clinics Network – a joint initiative between Care Services Improvement Partnership (CSIP) North West and the Royal College of Psychiatrists, with contributions from users, carers and other relevant disciplines and agencies. The Memory Services National Accreditation Process is now expanding to provide accreditation for memory clinic services countrywide.

It is hoped that this will continue to evolve and to support standards which enable positive management of the transition to dementia and the delivery of a full range of psychosocial interventions as well as current and future pharmacological treatments.

Dementia in combination with other common mental health conditions

The presentation of late-life depression and anxiety in conjunction with cognitive impairment and consequent difficulties for diagnosis are well known. This is acknowledged in the *National Service Framework for Older People* (Department of Health 2001) and the National Institute for Health and Clinical Excellence/Social Care Institute for Excellence (2006) *Dementia clinical practice guideline 42*. The latter reviews both psychological and pharmacological interventions for depression and anxiety and recommends that: 'cognitive behavioural therapy, which may involve the active participation of their carers, may be considered as part of treatment'. The Guidance makes no specific reference to adaptations or assessments that might be necessary to enable delivery of the first mentioned treatment – stating simply that cognitive behavioural therapy (CBT) is a 'recognised treatment for depression and anxiety in general use, and mental health professionals from various disciplines may be trained in its use'. They also suggest a range of other interventions, such as 'reminiscence therapy, multisensory stimulation, animal assisted therapy and exercise', and antidepressant medication for major depressive disorder (National Institute for Health and Clinical Excellence/Social Care Institute for Excellence 2006: 278).

Laidlaw *et al.* (2003) describe adaptations for the use of CBT with older people and a number of studies applying this with people with depression and dementia. These interventions emphasise the behavioural elements of CBT strategies: increasing pleasant events or problem-solving; both involving caregivers extensively. The authors also describe indirect approaches, working primarily with caregivers to reduce their stress and, it is hoped, result in improved care and associated benefits for the person with dementia, thus developing a positive cycle with further improvements in the carers' levels of distress (Laidlaw *et al.* 2003: 144–45).

In addition, Alexopoulos and his co-workers (Alexopoulos *et al.* 2002) have described a sub-group of older people with depression, whose symptoms are characterised by 'cognitive or executive functioning deficits and psychomotor retardation' (p. 98). Though not replicated in all studies (Butters *et al.* 2004), there is evidence that people with this depression variant show a poor response to usual antidepressant drug treatment (Potter *et al.* 2004, Alexopoulos *et al.* 2004, 2005). The PROSPECT Study, a US trial, comparing algorithm-based care for depression in older people with usual care (Bogner *et al.* 2007: 926), found that depressed older adults with executive dysfunction have low remission and response rates to 'usual care, but benefit from collaborative primary care and depression care management'. Problem solving therapy (PST) targeting the concrete behavioural deficits of older people with depression with executive dysfunction has been shown to be effective in addressing their specific clinical needs (Alexopoulos, Raue and Arean 2003, Alexopoulos *et al.* 2008).

Early stages of dementia and multidisciplinary teams

Early assessment and diagnosis of dementia is a complex challenge for multidisciplinary team working: no single profession's specialist skill holds the key to this process. In different individuals with dementia there is great variability in the early stage changes in cognition, behaviour and personality. These then overlap in a complex way with other mental health conditions and normal ageing. Even when assessments are reviewed together with evidence from brain imaging, the picture may be far from clear. Changes arising from the early stages of dementia are then further complicated by the person's physical health, history, their response to the condition and that of their family. All the foregoing make it particularly critical that different disciplines work effectively together to review and weigh evidence from their different methods of investigation and that they develop a good understanding and respect for their colleagues' work and skills. This is an essential building block from which personalised interventions can then be developed.

Terminology

> The term 'dementia' is used to describe a syndrome which may be caused by a number of illnesses, in which there is progressive decline in multiple areas of function, including decline in memory, reasoning, communication skills and the ability to carry out daily activities. Alongside this decline, individuals may develop behavioural and psychological symptoms such as depression, psychosis, aggression and wandering ...
>
> (Department of Health 2009a: 15)

Local demographic picture

The City of Salford is an urban district within the Greater Manchester conurbation, with a population of approximately 219,200, of whom approximately 39,600 are over the age of 65 years.

The area is predominantly urban, with a small suburban 'fringe'. In terms of Indices of Multiple Deprivation, the average score for Salford is 36.51, placing the City as the 15th most deprived out of 354 local authorities in England. As a whole, the population has significantly worse health than the national average on 24 out of 32 key indicators (Association of Public Health Observatories and Department of Health 2009). These include some of the highest rates for alcohol misuse, smoking, heart disease, stroke, and for over 65s 'not in good health'. As a result, vascular dementias also occur at a higher frequency than for the population of England and Wales as a whole.

About Salford older people's services

Mental health services for older people in Salford have been separate from working age provision since the early 1980s, and have involved a range of disciplines in regular liaison with Salford Community and Social Services. However, organisation of health and social services staff into formal integrated older people's community mental health teams (CMHTs), with unitary bases and line management, only occurred in 2007. Community Psychiatric Nurses (CPNs) make up the largest group of professionals within each team, with STR (Support Time and Recovery) workers, occupational therapy (OT), clinical psychology, social work and psychiatry in smaller proportions.

A separate memory clinic service – the Memory Assessment and Treatment Service (MATS) – was instigated in 2005. Like many others, it was funded by local Primary Care Trust commissioners in the wake of the first National Institute for Health and Clinical Excellence (2001) *Technology Appraisal TA19*. Thus initial funding focused on dementia assessment and diagnosis and treatment of 100 individuals with Alzheimer's disease. Referrals grew rapidly in the first few years, but further developments were delayed by the extended process of consultation around the revised National Institute for Health and Clinical Excellence (2007) *Technology Appraisal 111*.

Subsequent bids for increased funding – incorporating service re-design to optimise team capacity – were successful in 2008, at which time the referral rate exceeded 400 per annum. At the time of writing (January 2010), referrals continue to grow with more people now referred in the earlier stages of dementia. The team attempts to respond to escalating demand through continual review of practice. MATS has moved from a traditional consultant-led model to a fully multidisciplinary approach, with nursing and OT leading initial assessment and monitoring. Part-time psychiatry and psychology staff contribute mainly through multidisciplinary consultation and targeted involvement at appropriate stages of assessment and treatment on the basis of agreed pathways.

All referrals for older people's CMHTs and MATS services are received at a Single Entry Point. The CMHTs operate a duty system for initial and urgent assessments, combined with an allocation meeting to discuss referrals, identify care co-ordinators and appropriate clinicians to progress assessment and treatment within the Care Programme Approach (CPA). Referrals for investigation and diagnosis of possible mild to moderate dementias without challenging behaviours are allocated to the MATS service. Older people's CMHTs manage complex dementia with challenging behaviours.

This chapter will use three brief case studies to explore issues around the diagnosis and management of mild cognitive impairment and early to moderate stages of dementia, together with associated anxiety and depression. The cases also reflect different stages in the development of MATS and older people's CMHT services. Some implications for multidisciplinary practice and service design will also be considered.

Case study 1

Mr D, a 71-year-old married man, was referred to the single point of entry for older adult mental health services. Mr D's concern was of slowly deteriorating memory. Some years earlier he had been referred to working age adult mental health services with depression and reports of memory problems, but there was no other mental health history.

The CMHT duty officer felt a referral to the then recently established MATS team would be most in keeping with Mr D's needs. At this time initial assessment was undertaken by the team psychiatrist.

Initial assessment

Mr D's first involvement with mental health services had been six years earlier. At the time, he reported depression and had also complained of poor memory. From the records available it was unclear if his memory concerns were considered at that time. He had been prescribed an antidepressant but had no further investigations or involvement with mental health services. In retrospect, it remained unclear whether these initial memory problems were related to low mood or were symptomatic of early signs of a developing organic condition.

Mr D was married with no children and had been retired since the age of 65. He had undergone major cardiac surgery in 1993 and been fitted with a pacemaker. There was a family history of dementia: Mr D had lost his mother to dementia some four years earlier.

The psychiatrist noted a moderate degree of depression, but also felt there might be an underlying organic process. He prescribed antidepressant medication, and requested further neuropsychological assessment (from LH) and neuro-imaging investigations. Mr D was referred for both MRI and Serial Positron Emission Computed Tomography. The former uses a strong magnetic field within which molecules align themselves. When the field is removed these give up energy which can be translated into an image, revealing even small degrees of damage to the brain. The latter produces images of cerebral blood flow, and as such is a functional rather than an anatomical imaging technique.

Psychological assessment

Mr D was assessed at home, at times in the presence of his wife in order to corroborate some of the information that he provided. Mr D reported that he had been feeling 'fed up' for some time and was becoming increasingly concerned about his failing memory. This concern was exacerbated by his awareness that his mother had suffered a dementia syndrome. Mr D's insight into his problems was variable and he tended to strive to present a capable social front.

Mr D was able to recall and to speak with relative ease about many aspects of his past. According to Mr D, he had worked in the building trade as a contractual engineer throughout his working life. He was used to being organized and pragmatic. Due to the demands of his job, he had spent significant amounts of time away from home over the past 35 years and was still finding it difficult to adjust to life post retirement.

Mr and Mrs D had not had any children of their own and their social network was minimal. Mr D had not retained any friends from work and Mrs D occasionally kept company with her sister and nieces. By and large, however, his retirement meant that, for the first time in their marriage, they spent most of their time in each other's company. Although he found it difficult to articulate this, it was clear that this significant increase in time spent with his wife was a contributory factor to Mr D's low mood.

Mr D's wife was also seen separately from her husband. From her report, it was clear that Mr D was becoming increasingly disorientated in time and place. As a result he was becoming increasingly intolerant of his problems and more and more abrupt with his wife. Pre-existing marital tension was now being amplified by Mr D's cognitive condition and the extent to which he was relying upon his wife to meet his every need. According to Mrs D, her husband had always expected her to perform a traditional role within the relationship and since his retirement this expectation had grown stronger. His failing memory and associated low mood were placing increasing demands upon Mrs D, both to perform more of the household chores and for her needs to come second to those of her husband.

Neuropsychological assessment

Neuropsychological assessment was planned to determine the extent of Mr D's cognitive impairment. It was clear from initial discussions that he was experiencing some expressive language problems in addition to his more obvious memory impairment. The cognitive screening element of the Cambridge Examination for Mental Disorders in the Elderly – Revised was completed: the Cambridge Cognitive Examination for Mental Disorders – Revised (CAMCOG-R; Roth *et al.* 1988). However, the extent of

Mr D's distress was such that it was thought prudent to draw initial conclusions from this and not to pursue further formal assessment at this time.

The screening assessment confirmed mild cognitive impairment, with specific difficulties due to poor orientation to time and place and difficulty processing abstract concepts. It was also apparent that compensatory strategies employed by Mrs D to reduce her husband's frustration at his poor recall were disguising the extent of his memory problems. Whilst this was done with good intent, at times it prevented Mr D from exercising his remaining capacity, and in turn exacerbated his symptoms.

Scan results and feedback

The scans suggested atrophy in the temporal and parietal lobes of Mr D's brain. This was consistent with the screening test results and with a diagnosis of dementia of the Alzheimer's type, although some generalized patchy perfusion was also noted which could indicate co-existing cerebro-vascular disease. The psychiatrist felt that a trial of anti-dementia medication could be initiated. Since the psychologist had been able to establish a therapeutic dialogue with the couple, it was felt that a joint approach would help the couple understand the diagnosis within the context of their respective lives. Psychological management would be needed to address the interaction of marital tensions and dementia symptoms.

The psychiatrist and psychologist met with Mr and Mrs D to explain the test results and diagnosis and to answer any immediate questions. It was also agreed that Mr D would receive on-going support and review from a CPN to monitor the anti-dementia medication and the antidepressant medication already prescribed.

The role of the psychologist

The psychologist remained involved, in order to support and advise Mr and Mrs D during this difficult period. At this time, the psychologist's role was seen as two-fold: the delivery of a needs-based psychological intervention for the complex dementia and marital issues; and facilitation of a co-ordinated transition into the relevant support services.

Generally, the period since referral had been characterized by stability in Mr D's condition, but it was punctuated by periods of increased distress, marital tension and increasingly problematic behavioural issues. During this time the psychologist's role has covered:

- Helping the client and his wife understand and adjust to the diagnosis and its effect on their lives as changes from the condition evolve.
- Advising the couple on how to best manage specific issues such as risk, confusion and disorientation.
- Encouraging Mrs D to access services for dementia carers.

Supporting Mr D with his diagnosis

In the initial months following diagnosis, Mr D was provided with advice, information about his condition, encouragement and practical strategies to best utilize his cognitive strengths. At times he demonstrated insight into the extent of his problems and their impact. Memory aids and plans were developed in tandem with Mrs D who provided much of the insight into Mr D's memory function and its effect on his mood. This common cause of frustration for both Mr and Mrs D often led to arguments and distress. The work of the psychologist at these times often drew more on marital therapy and relationship counselling strategies than on cognitive behavioural interventions for memory problems arising from dementia.

Supporting Mrs D as she acquired the role of carer

Initially, the psychologist often acted as an advocate on behalf of Mr D in discussions with his wife. As is often the case in dementia care, Mrs D tried to work out whether Mr D was behaving in a certain way because of his organic impairment or because of his personality and existing patterns of behaviour: a search that is often ultimately misguided and futile. However, it also indicated the confusion that Mrs D sometimes experienced regarding the manifestations of her husband's condition (see also Quinn *et al.* 2008). The clinician's role at these times morphed from being one of educator (helping Mrs D understand the anomalies, contradictions, inconsistencies and curiosities of dementia) to one of listener and ally.

At times of heightened distress, Mrs D would express her concerns and emotions, and need help to process her regret, loss, anger, resentment, isolation and burden, despite still loving and caring for her husband. These sessions often bore witness to the underlying marital conflicts that pre-dated the onset of Mr D's diagnosis. It was as a consequence of these discussions with Mrs D that she began to accept the possible benefits of accessing and utilizing care support networks. Whilst this meant that she had to begin to identify aspects of herself with the role of carer, she came to recognize that she could no longer 'walk this path alone' and that it might help to share her experiences with others in the same predicament.

Education

As Mr D's symptoms worsened he began to lose things more frequently and to develop elaborate stories in order to explain these losses. This response was understandable and rational when perceived from his increasingly confused and potentially suspicious perspective. However, Mrs D's initial response was to correct Mr D and try to 'talk him into accepting the truth'. This triggered arguments, angry scenes and distress. The psychologist used a solution-focused narrative to help her understand Mr D's 'stories' (no matter how elaborate), and to change her response from confrontation and challenge to acceptance and resolution of the emotion associated with Mr D's reactions (validation therapy). Again, the role was of educator and informed ally, enabling Mrs D to become 'expert' and thus experience a relative improvement in her feelings of control over a very frightening and debilitating situation.

Signposting to services

At the point at which he relinquished his driving licence, the relationship between Mr D and his wife had changed. She became the driver, a role that Mr D had restricted throughout their marriage. Not only did this serve to highlight the chronicity of their marital discord but it also drew attention to the amount of isolation Mr D was experiencing. He accepted a referral to a voluntary agency which provided him with a befriender, whose task it was to join Mr D on walks to local parks and areas of interest. This helped to reduce the burden placed on Mrs D as the sole provider of safe activity outside the home, but unfortunately it proved time-limited due to logistical changes within the voluntary agency.

Accessing respite care

The clinician, at this point, identified and facilitated a respite care placement for Mr D. Continuing subtle encouragement was given regarding this to both Mr and Mrs D, who had their own independent concerns about its potential costs and benefits.

Reflections

At the time of writing, the psychologist remains in contact with Mr and Mrs D. A reality of his involvement during much of this period has been that the psychologist has been the key professional involved whose role enabled him to support this couple long term. An overwhelming point of concern for Mrs D has been how to make sense of and to contact all the people and agencies involved in providing services at different times. Having established a key role in understanding the dynamics of their marriage and the impact of Mr D's dementia, it has fallen to the psychologist to act as the common denominator that connects the different elements of mental health services, primary care, voluntary agencies and social services. There are a wide range of specific clinical interventions that a psychologist can offer for complex and chronic organic conditions and that have been provided in this instance. Yet it may be that this case most exemplifies the importance of continuity of care, delivered within the context of an holistic understanding of the person with dementia, their life history and personal relationships.

Case study 2

Mrs S, a 73-year-old, widowed for just over two years, had become increasingly anxious in the home she had shared with her husband. She told family and friends that this was because, as a non-driver, it was more difficult for her to get out and about. Six months before referral she had moved to a housing association flat in the same locality, but closer to her son and his family. Mrs S had seemed particularly anxious after the move and despite their proximity, lacked confidence going out to shops alone. This had improved, but she remained anxious, avoided old friends, became flustered by anything new and was unusually forgetful. The general practitioner (GP) had followed the local pre-referral medical screening protocol, including undertaking relevant blood tests. Finding no medically treatable explanation, he had referred her to MATS.

Initial assessment

Mrs S was invited to attend for assessment using a choose-and-book process, during which the benefits of attending accompanied by a relative or friend who could provide additional information about her difficulties were emphasised.

Mrs S attended accompanied by her son. They were seen for initial assessment: semi-structured interview and client and carer assessments, undertaken by a CPN and OT, respectively. The interview was based on the available literature on good practice in

Table 7.1 Possible screening tools for mood and anxiety

Assessment tool	Rationale for use and authors
Geriatric Depression Scale – short form (GDS)	Well-established depression scale designed for use with older people (Yesavage *et al.* 1983)
Hospital Anxiety and Depression Scale (HADS)	Not specifically designed for use with older people, but can be useful for assessment of anxiety in older people with mild cognitive impairment or early dementia (Zigmond and Snaith 1983)
General Health Questionnaire (GHQ-28)	A scaleable version of the well-established measure of clinically significant distress (Goldberg and Hillier 1979)

assessment for dementia diagnosis and developed by the MATS' nurse and OT leads (NB and GS, respectively). It covered:

- Pre-diagnostic counselling issues (see Marzanski 2000, Elson 2007).
- Consent and capacity.
- Team confidentiality, record keeping, access to records, etc.
- General and medical histories, including any contraindications for MRI scan.
- Presenting difficulties.
- Current functional performance in Activities of Daily Living.
- Current risks, including driving status.

The client assessment consisted of:

- Mini-mental State Examination (MMSE; Folstein, Folstein and McHugh 1975). Standardised version of the well-established screening test for dementia (Malloy and Standish 1997).
- DemTect (Kalbe *et al.* 2004). This brief measure is acceptable to clients, and has been shown to have greater specificity and sensitivity in the detection of mild cognitive impairment and early dementia in well-functioning individuals (Larner 2007). It was administered because the client had scored relatively highly on the MMSE.
- A mood and anxiety scale, where appropriate (see Table 7.1).

The carer assessment included completion of the:

- Bristol Activities of Daily Living Scale (Bucks *et al.* 1996).
- Carer stress measure (where appropriate).

Key findings from the assessment

The pre-diagnostic counselling was designed to ensure that Mrs S understood the reason for assessment and consented to the process. She was fully aware that her referral might lead to a diagnosis of some form of dementia. She disclosed that she had been frightened of this for some time:

> It's been weighing on my mind and I'm going from bad to worse [she had not wanted to talk about the issue] but my son winkled it out of me. He said, 'Mum,

we should get you checked – what if something can be done? You shouldn't miss out'. After it came out with him I felt relieved but then panicky – I thought what if I have? What will they all think? I wouldn't let him tell [daughter-in-law] or my girls. Who wants to spend time with a mad old person? How will I manage? I've always been the person people can rely on.

Mrs S's MMSE and DemTect scores were relatively high. Her manner during interview and the Hospital Anxiety and Depression Scale (Zigmond and Snaith 1983) score also showed that she had a clinically significant level of anxiety. The nurse thought it possible that the lost marks on MMSE and DemTect might be attributable to this anxiety. According to her son, Mrs S had not been prone to anxiety until recently and had coped with many difficult events throughout her life. The information provided by the client and her son was consistent in identifying changes in her abilities over the last 18 months.

The next stages of the process were then explained to Mrs S and her son. The initial assessment would be discussed at the MDT meeting the following day. Mrs S's high scores, very mild level of cognitive impairment and anxiety met the team's criteria for further assessment by the psychologist and for review of scan choice with the team psychiatrist. Mrs S agreed to attend for a brain scan, and to meet the psychologist who would undertake additional cognitive assessments and review Mrs S's feelings of anxiety.

Neuropsychological assessment

Mrs S was assessed using a brief screening battery of tests which could be supplemented by further tests if necessary. The psychologist (RD) had developed this on the basis of the neuropsychological literature, the need to target a limited assessment resource to unclear or complex cases and to minimise stress for the client. The detailed initial assessment meant that the psychologist was able to avoid duplicating questions about general history and to focus on specific details (see Table 7.2).

The psychologist considered the test results carefully in the context of this lady's marked anxiety. However, given the overall pattern of scores, it was clear that Mrs S

Table 7.2 Neuropsychological screening tests

Assessment tool	Rationale for use and authors
CAMCOG-R	General cognitive screening instrument, which can also help identify areas of impairment for more detailed testing (Roth *et al.* 1988)
Wechsler (WTAR)	Indicates pre-morbid ability level (Wechsler 2001)
Wechsler Adult Intelligence Scale (WAIS-III UK)	Similarities, Block Design and Symbol Search – sub-tests selected for general relevance to dementia assessment from the well-known and standardised test (Wechsler 1999)
Wechsler Memory Scale – 3rd Edition (WMS-III UK)	Logical Memory, Visual Reproduction, Word Lists and Digit Span – sub-tests exploring verbal and visual memory, (both recall and recognition) and working memory (Wechsler 1997)
Behavioural Assessment of Dysexecutive Syndrome (BADS)	Key Search sub-test selected from this battery of tests designed for assessment of executive functioning (Wilson *et al.* 1996)
Delis-Kaplan Executive Function System (D-KEFS)	Sub-tests selected from this test system designed for assessment of executive functioning (Delis *et al.* 2001)

was no longer functioning at a level consistent with her age and estimates of her pre-morbid IQ. The psychologist felt that anxiety was adding to her difficulties, but that this was in response to an underlying cognitive decline.

Mrs S also disclosed more of her fears about dementia. Throughout her life she had prided herself on her competence at work and as a wife and mother. Mrs S was aware that she was becoming forgetful, and frustrated that she made 'stupid, stupid mistakes' with baking and other complex tasks. 'I'm so slow now. I have to check and check'. She kept a careful diary of events, to which she would refer when friends or family rang, to 'hold up her end' in the conversation as usual. Mrs S had avoided meeting friends face-to-face, when she could not use her diary and feared that she would be 'completely caught out'.

Brain scan

Findings from the MRI brain scan showed no evidence of significant vascular changes but there were some changes to the temporal and parietal lobes which could be consistent with early stages of Alzheimer's disease.

Multidisciplinary review

The initial assessment, brain scan and neuropsychological tests results were reviewed by the team during their weekly clinical meeting. The combination of results confirmed that Mrs S's difficulties were not attributable to anxiety alone, but were consistent with the early stages of Alzheimer's disease. Any vascular component was thought to be mild. It was noted that Mrs S had stated her wish to be told the diagnosis, and for information to be shared with her son.

The team considered other issues, including the possibility that diagnosis might trigger deterioration in Mrs S's already high level of anxiety. Options for anxiety management and psychosocial intervention were reviewed with the psychologist. The latter had noted that much of Mrs S's anxiety and changed behaviour related to her uncertainty about how she might be affected by the condition and her anxieties about other people's reactions to her difficulties. An individual anxiety management approach could be offered, but there would be a delay as the psychologist had a waiting list at that time. Participation in a supportive group (which included some general stress management) was considered a useful step as it might also help address her feeling of isolation. The psychologist suggested that Mrs S might respond well to an occupational therapy approach to management of the practical difficulties arising from her cognitive impairment. The psychiatrist reviewed Mrs S's electrocardiogram results and decided that a trial of AChEIs should be offered.

The nurse arranged a joint meeting with the team psychiatrist, Mrs S and her family to begin the process of sharing the diagnosis, to discuss options for treatment and negotiate a mutually agreed plan.

Occupational therapy assessment and intervention

Graff *et al.* (2006, 2007) and Bennet and Liddle (2008) have described effective OT interventions in memory clinic and community dementia care. Drawing on this and other evidence-based practice, the OT undertook a detailed home-based activity analysis of Mrs S's current functional performance in those activities of daily living that she had described as affected: offering guests hot drinks; using familiar routines to store items in, and using the central heating system. Generally, Mrs S was coping well, except with more complex tasks, when she felt rushed, or needed to remember multiple pieces of information, such as when offering tea to several family members or neighbours.

Formulation and plan

The functional assessments indicated deficits in the initiation and planning stages of each activity affecting her ability to independently carry out the task. With careful consideration to practical compensatory strategies to overcome these deficits, the OT was able to identify a method of intervention that would enable Mrs S to continue completing her identified activities independently. A period of weekly therapy sessions followed, offering repetitive rehearsal of the strategies. Mrs S proved to be highly motivated to find ways to continue to cope independently. The OT worked with her to further develop the written instruction strategies Mrs S already used to 'cover-up' her difficulties. They developed detailed step-by-step reminders for essential tasks – such as managing the central heating controls. 'Flash cards' were made to help Mrs S remember family preferences for drinks when they visited and visual cues were developed to help her find and store things in her kitchen cupboards. Each element was introduced sequentially as part of a clear written plan. Success with these increased Mrs S's confidence in having family and friends to visit and, in turn, her anxiety and mood improved. Mrs S made considerable strides quite quickly, as she proved highly motivated and used her systems diligently.

Further intervention

The team felt that Mrs S had made some progress in her adjustment to the diagnosis but was still distressed – she scored a clinically significant 8 on the GHQ-28. This was discussed with her by the team psychologist, who also explained options for a brief anxiety management programme or group support. Mrs S felt that she would like the opportunity to talk about her experiences with other people 'who could laugh because they were doing the same things – not just be sorry for me', and opted to attend a group run by the team. This offered an opportunity for people with early stages of dementia to explore their experience and ways of coping within a supportive peer group. The group was not open to carers; they could access a range of other groups and interventions locally.

Support group for people with the early stages of Alzheimer's disease

The team had developed a programme specifically targeted to the needs of people with early stage Alzheimer's disease. Meetings were held at a local non-NHS community facility which offered a relaxed meeting place in a non-stigmatising environment. A brief outline of session content is contained in Table 7.3.

A psychology assistant visited participants at home after conclusion of the group to complete standardised assessments of well-being and to evaluate the effectiveness of the group using a simple questionnaire. Carers were also asked for their views as to whether the group had had any impact on the person with dementia.

Following the group, Mrs S's GHQ-28 score had dropped to the point that it was no longer clinically significant. She felt that she understood more about her Alzheimer's disease and was more able to admit her difficulties to others. She also felt that the group

Table 7.3 Group for people with early stages of Alzheimer's disease

Session 1	Introductions, planning future sessions
Session 2	What is Alzheimer's disease? What is memory? Drugs for Alzheimer's disease
Session 3	Coping with memory loss
Session 4	Life roles and changes, staying positive and local resources
Session 5	Exercise, diet, stress and relaxation
Session 6	Life planning and advanced directives
Session 7	Final review meeting and planning peer support meetings

had shared her values: wanting to continue with an active life for as long as possible, challenging negative stereotypes of the condition. After some thought and discussion with the group facilitators, Mrs S had 'taken courage' and disclosed her diagnosis to two of her closest friends. They had helped challenge her fears by proving supportive, understanding and actively continuing their friendship. Mrs S's daughter-in-law also reported:

> I noticed she was always bubbly and cheerful when I picked her up after the sessions ... [she] told me bits about the group and what they've talked about. I don't think there has been any change in how her memory is ... but she has come away full of enthusiasm, which does carry over for a day or two.

Outcome

Eighteen months after Mrs S's initial visit to MATS, she was still coping independently at home. OT assessment identified some decline in her ability to undertake more complex activities of daily living. For example, her son helped her check through her finances on a frequent basis; he and her daughter-in-law now kept a copy of her diary and helped monitor key appointments; they helped her plan and undertake her 'big shop' at the supermarket.

It was notable that she had progressed to the point that she could acknowledge her problem and share her diagnosis with family and selected close friends, though she was also, possibly realistically, wary of sharing this more widely. She was keen to live as positively with the diagnosis as possible and to take up any options for support or treatment. She continued to be a regular attendee at informal follow-up support sessions.

Reflections

The reaction of Mrs S to her developing cognitive loss reflects the sense of stigma still attached to dementia, and the very real rejection many people experience from others in their family and social circle. This was an important contributory factor to her anxiety and isolation. Apart from the element of peer support, a direct benefit of attendance at the early stages group was that it also provided a natural opportunity for her to make some 'cognitive-behavioural experiments' which challenged some of her beliefs and fears about dementia without resort to formal therapy. Help to plan how and when to share diagnosis improved the chances that her experience would be positive, and not one of rejection. Sadly, many people are still referred for first assessment at much later stages, when their capacity to benefit from early interventions and to participate in planning for their futures are much restricted.

Case study 3

Mrs F had undergone surgery and in-patient treatment. At out-patient follow-up she had been identified as depressed by the Hospital Consultant. She was prescribed anti-depressants and referred to a generic psychological therapies service. Following trial of a brief psychological intervention, the therapist felt that Mrs F was 'not psychologically-minded … [and] unable to make progress'. He wrote to the GP suggesting that given Mrs F's age (76 years) she be referred to the older people's CMHT for a psychiatric assessment and review of medication options.

Initial assessment

Initially, Mrs F was seen by a CPN for further assessment, together with her husband and a daughter who lived locally. They said that Mrs F had become progressively more depressed over the last six months, had gradually stopped undertaking her usual household tasks, and was spending most of her time 'just sitting' in a chair, with the television on. Her family were all concerned and had tried to get her to 'snap out of it'. At times Mrs F would seem 'more like her usual self' (for example during a family holiday), but this was unpredictable. The change was having a secondary impact on the daughter, who had been leaving her youngest son with his grandparents two evenings a week to enable her to work. Mr F, who had become the principle childminder, taking the boy to football practice, etc., was finding this increasingly difficult as he took over household activities from his wife.

Initial treatments with antidepressants and CBT had not proved successful. Mrs F had been unable to engage with the process of identifying negative cognitions or generating alternatives. She had not found this therapy helpful. She had tried the anti-depressants, but found the side effects difficult, and on careful questioning admitted that she 'didn't like medication' and so had taken them erratically. The husband was now presenting as increasingly distressed and frustrated by the impact of his wife's depression on their lives.

CPN intervention

The CPN noted that Mrs F's depression had followed a very stressful period, with multiple episodes of ill-health, which might be sufficient to explain the onset of depression. He also felt that Mrs F and the family had not had sufficient understanding about how the medication worked, so there had not been an effective trial of anti-depressants. Following review with the psychiatrist, a medication plan was agreed and explained in detail to the family, together with the importance of taking the medication as prescribed. The CPN would visit to monitor progress and advise about side effects and other problems.

Following an appropriate trial period, the CPN reported back to the psychiatrist that medication appeared to be having little effect on Mrs F's mood, but noted also that she showed fewer overt signs of sadness or tearfulness than the CPN would normally expect. Her predominant presentation was of apathy – loss of her usual 'get up and go'. Mrs F herself agreed that this was the case: she just 'didn't feel like doing anything' and kept hoping to wake up one day with her old enthusiasm for life.

The CPN and psychiatrist reviewed the case, and felt that little more would be gained by further trials of medication and speculated that some mild cognitive impairment might be responsible for her symptoms. A referral was made for psychological review of options for assessment and intervention.

Psychological assessment

Mrs F was not positive about the referral. She felt that her previous contact with psychological therapy had been 'no help at all' and, if anything, had made her feel even more despondent. However, she reluctantly agreed to an appointment and was seen by the older people's CMHT psychologist, together with her husband and daughter who had attended due to the family's concern about lack of progress. Mrs F was asked whether she would prefer to be seen alone, but stated that she was happy for the other members of the family to be present. The psychologist agreed to this, as the service took an inclusive approach to involving family in assessments. However, although a majority of questions were addressed to Mrs F, she said very little, with Mr F and his daughter dominating the discussion.

The psychologist was struck by the accounts of Mrs F and her family about her difficulties and by the level of stress in the family as a whole. There appeared to be a marked reduction and slowing compared with Mrs F's previous level of activity, some of which could be directly attributable to her changed health status. The family also described her as being changed in personality. She had experienced more than 20 years of ill-health, but had coped with cheerfulness and energy. From an assertive, competent woman, she now did little unless prompted 'and nagged' to do so. She did not seem deeply distressed, was seldom tearful and reported few overtly depressed thoughts. She and the family all agreed that she 'didn't feel like doing anything' and 'nothing was interesting any more – it was all too much effort'.

The psychologist felt that it would be important to see Mrs F on her own. However, it continued to be difficult to get much information: her answers were very brief and she never expanded upon any response unless prompted. Generally the main impression was of her loss of interest and energy and that she also felt nagged at by the family. She appeared well-orientated and informed about current events, but occasionally seemed to have difficulty recalling the sequencing of complex events around her recent history and medical treatment.

The psychologist was struck by the marked changes in executive skills and behaviour reported by Mrs F and her family, which might also be consistent with a depression with co-existing cognitive changes. A short screening assessment of Mrs F's cognition was undertaken (see Table 7.2, earlier), in addition to repeating standard depression measures. The psychologist explained the rationale for this to Mrs F and her husband as follows:

- The psychiatrist and CPN had done a thorough job of trying antidepressant medication. This had not worked.
- Anyone who is depressed may not be thinking as efficiently as normal, but some depression in older people may be accompanied by changes in thinking patterns, which can be shown up by standard 'psychometric' tests.
- There are reports that these forms of depression may be more resistant to antidepressant medication.

The psychologist explained what the tests would entail, and arranged for these to be undertaken over the next few weeks.

Neuropsychological assessment

Mrs F showed very mild signs of general cognitive impairment based on the CAMCOG-R (Roth *et al.*1988). However, her scores on tests sensitive to executive functioning deficits were consistent with reports of the depression-executive dysfunction syndrome (Lockwood, Alexopoulos and van Gorp 2002). The psychologist explained the test results to Mrs F and her husband, and supplied them with a brief report in lay terms to explain key findings and recommendations to help manage her symptoms. An objective of this approach was to begin to change the attributions of Mrs F and her family about her condition and their expectations for her future functioning, whilst also maintaining therapeutic optimism that improvement was possible. The benefits of taking a behavioural problem solving approach, and of introducing plans at a slow pace, to avoid 'overloading' her were explained. The role for family in providing moral support for Mrs F was emphasised. Consistency was also provided by the psychiatrist and CPN in reiterating this explanation and supporting the new approach.

Under guidance from the psychologist, an assistant worked with Mrs F and her family to set specific goals to build up her activities within simple daily routines and to introduce some brief regular enjoyable activities outside the home. The importance of making slow, modest changes, and not trying for too many changes was also stressed. Progress was monitored through a combination of home visits and telephone checks. There was a major shift in the family's interactions with Mrs F. Her husband began to express less frustration, and spoke positively about small changes that the couple managed to achieve. He also began to acknowledge his own need to adapt his activities and expectations to his own level of energy. The couple negotiated occasional breaks from child minding with their daughter and booked a few inexpensive short breaks – 'to give us both a rest from daily chores'.

Reflections

The team were very open with Mrs F and her family about their own process of assessment and, having settled upon a treatment strategy, also attempted to provide consistency in terms of explanations and approach across all disciplines. The emphasis placed by the team on developing a shared explanation of her difficulties with Mrs F and her family was important in addressing their attributions about her condition and developing their commitment and confidence in trying new strategies after the initial failures. The behavioural approach used drew on the general goal planning and problem solving literature, as well as the PST approach used by Alexopoulos *et al.* (2008). The practical, concrete nature of this strategy was also easy for Mrs F and her family to understand and directly tackled their own concerns.

This case also illustrated the importance of effective contacts and processes between CMHTs, memory assessment and other later life services – an area for continuing attention if the needs are to be met of people whose difficulties straddle the criteria for more than one service.

Discussion

It is probable that in addition to the assessments and interventions used, various team characteristics were important in achieving change in the examples described. Unlike the generic and working age services, the older adult service was experienced in working with older people and understood the particular risks of adopting a narrow diagnosis-based choice of standardised treatment packages. Important elements influencing outcome included emphasising the following:

- A pre-diagnostic counselling approach at initial contact with memory services, and incorporation of each person's choices around diagnosis.
- Understanding the person's whole history.
- Including family members in assessment and treatment plans.
- Considering the possibility of specific mild cognitive impairment complicating other mental health presentations and vice versa.
- Utilising more active, behavioural strategies of intervention.
- Involving the skills of a range of disciplines.

The first and third case examples illustrate the delays, stress and demoralisation experienced by people with later life problems and their families when assessment and treatment is ill-informed about their needs. These initial problems also meant that the teams had the additional task of addressing earlier treatment failures to ensure the engagement of the clients and their families.

Documents such as the *National Service Framework for Older People* (Department of Health 2001) and *Everybody's Business* (Department of Health and Care Service Improvement Partnership 2005) have drawn attention to the need to end age discrimination and make services open to all people on the basis of need, not age. There is much debate about the best way to reduce stigmatisation and to deliver non-discriminatory mental health services to older people. Some have advocated opening services to all ages and the removal of specialist services. However, this is not always accompanied by a parallel recognition of the need for specialist skills and to re-engineer services to ensure that they in turn do not introduce new forms of discrimination by assuming a 'one size fits all' approach. Minshull (2007) provides a useful key summary of some of the dilemmas and issues to be addressed in delivering age inclusive services. More recently the documents: *A collective responsibility to act now on ageing and mental health* (Mental Health and Older People Forum 2008) and *New Horizons: A shared vision for mental health* (Department of Health 2009b) have acknowledged the complex issues involved in balancing the need for specialist practitioners and services with efforts to end age discrimination.

Irrespective of service model, there are other important issues to be addressed: generic and working age services need greater understanding of the assessment and care of people with early onset and in the early stages of dementia and effective pathways to ensure that their needs are met. There is a clear responsibility for specialist later life practitioners and services to contribute to this process.

The Salford MATS team has evolved gradually since its inception. Many of these changes have been dependent on the team's enthusiasm and commitment to their clients, their growing understanding of each other's roles and team skills development. The move to nursing and OT undertaking initial assessments was a key development. It followed a comprehensive piece of work systematising the assessment as a semi-structured interview and also helped establish a willingness in all team members to run simple 'PDSA' cycles to try out new options to deliver assessment and treatment more effectively.

At the outset of the service, a disproportionate element of the disclosure process fell on the team psychiatrists, whose role and time allocation to MATS made them most pressured to complete this work quickly. The active involvement of team members at all stages of assessment and planning means that the whole team are able to support the process of disclosure, information sharing and adjustment. They can work at the pace of the particular person with dementia and their carers.

There is potential to further develop the flexible model of practice used by the Salford MATS team and to learn from other services. For example, the Manchester Memory Clinic has demonstrated that specialist nurses can develop high levels of diagnostic accuracy such that 'in a significant number of cases the initial diagnosis of dementia could be the responsibility of specialist nurses' (Page *et al.* 2008: 32), which could also expedite signposting to subsequent care pathways, reduce waiting times before basic aspects of the diagnosis are shared, and ensure prompt access to benefit entitlements and services. A continual (and continuing) issue for MATS has been the need to adopt a pragmatic approach to maximise team resources. The team has taken an active approach to adopting new ways of working, but there are benefits and conflicts as a result. The Croydon Memory Service's evaluation of their changing practices in the next chapter of this book provides an interesting window into this experience.

Acknowledgements

The authors wish to thank Claire Matchwick and Laura Bettney, Psychology Assistants, for their respective contributions to neuropsychological testing, clinical interventions and the development and evaluation of the group for people with early stages of dementia.

References

Age Concern and the Mental Health Foundation (2006) *Promoting mental health and well-being in later-life: A first report of the UK inquiry into mental health and well-being in later life*, London: Age Concern and the Mental Health Foundation. Available: www.mhilli.org (accessed 4 February 2010).

———(2007) *Improving services and support for older people with mental health problems. The second report from the UK inquiry into mental health and well-being in later life*, London: Age Concern and the Mental Health Foundation. Available: www.mhilli.org/documents/Inquiryfinalreport-fullreport.pdf (accessed 4 February 2010).

Alexopoulos, G.S., Kiosses, D.N., Klimstra, S., Kalayam, B. and Buser, M.L. (2002) 'Clinical presentation of the 'depression-executive dysfunction syndrome' of later life', *American Journal of Geriatric Psychiatry*, 10: 98–106.

Alexopoulos, G.S., Kiosses, D.N., Murphy, C. and Heo, M. (2004) 'Executive dysfunction, heart disease burden, and remission of geriatric depression', *Neuropsychopharmacology*, 29: 2278–84.

Alexopoulos, G.S., Kiosses, D.N., Heo, M., Murphy, C.F., Shanmugham, B. and Gunning-Dixon, F. (2005) 'Executive dysfunction, and the course of geriatric depression', *Biological Psychiatry*, 58: 204–10.

Alexopoulos, G.S., Raue, P. and Arean, P. (2003) 'Problem-solving therapy versus supportive therapy in geriatric major depression with executive dysfunction', *American Journal of Geriatric Psychiatry*, 11: 46–52.

Alexopoulos, G.S., Raue, P.J., Kanellopoulos, D., Machin, S. and Arean, P. (2008) 'Problem-solving therapy versus supportive therapy for the depression-executive dysfunction syndrome of late life', *International Journal of Geriatric Psychiatry,* 23:782–88.

Alzheimer's Society (2007) *Dementia UK: A report into the prevalence and cost of Dementia, prepared by the Personal Social Services Research Unit (PSSRU) at the London School of Economics and the Institute of Psychiatry at King's College London for the Alzheimer's Society*, London: Alzheimer's Society.

Association of Public Health Observatories and Department of Health (2009) *Health Profile 2009: Salford*, London: Department of Health. Available: www.healthprofiles.info (accessed 4 February 2010).

Banerjee, S., Willis, R., Matthews, D., Contell, F., Chan, J. and Murray, J. (2007) 'Improving the quality of care for mild to moderate dementia: an evaluation of the Croydon Memory Service Model', *International Journal of Geriatric Psychiatry*, 22: 722–28.

Bennet, S. and Liddle, J. (2008) 'Community based Occupational Therapy improved daily functioning in people with dementia', *Australian Occupational Therapy Journal*, 55 (1): 73–74.

Bogner, H.R., Reynolds, C.F., Mulsant, B.H., Cary, M.S., Morales, K., Alexopoulos, G.S. and the PROSPECT Group (2007) 'The effects of memory, attention and executive dysfunction on outcomes of depression in a primary care intervention trial: the PROSPECT study', *International Journal of Geriatric Psychiatry*, 22: 922–29.

Bucks, R.S., Ashworth, D.L., Wilcock, G.K. and Siegfried, K. (1996) 'Assessment of activities of daily living: development of the Bristol Activities of Daily Living Scale', *Age and Ageing*, 25: 113–20.

Butters, M.A., Bhalla, R.K., Mulsant, B.H., Mazumdar, S., Houck, P.R., Begley, A.E., Dew, M.A., Pollock, B.G., Nebes, R.D., Becker, J.T. and Reynolds, C.F. (2004) 'Executive functioning, illness course, and relapse/recurrence in continuation and maintenance treatment of late-life depression. Is there a relationship?' *American Journal of Geriatric Psychiatry*, 12 (4): 387–94.

Charlesworth, G., Shepstone, L., Wilson, E., Reynolds, S., Mugford, M., Price, D., Harvey, I. and Poland, F. (2008) 'Befriending carers of people with dementia', *British Medical Journal*, 336 (7656): 1295–97.

Cheston, R., Jones, K. and Gilliard, J. (2003) 'Group psychotherapy and people with dementia', *Aging and Mental Health*, 7: 452–61.

Clare, L. (2003) 'Rehabilitation for people with dementia', in B.A. Wilson (ed.), *Neuropsychological rehabilitation theory and practice*, London: Taylor & Francis.

Clare, L. and Woods, R. (2004) 'Cognitive training and cognitive rehabilitation for people with early-stage Alzheimer's Disease: A review', *Neuropsychological Rehabilitation*, 14: 385–401.

Delis, D.C., Kaplan, E. and Kramer, J.H. (2001) *Delis-Kaplan Executive Function System (D-KEFS)*, Oxford: Pearson.

Department of Health (2001) *National Service Framework for Older People*, London: Department of Health.

——(2009a) *Living Well with Dementia: a National Dementia Strategy*, London: Department of Health.

——(2009b) *New Horizons: A shared vision for mental health*, London: Department of Health.

Department of Health and Care Service Improvement Partnership (2005) *Everybody's Business: Integrated Mental Health Services for Older Adults: A service development guide*, London: Department of Health. Available: www.everybodysbusiness.org.uk (accessed 4 February 2010).

Elson, P. (2007) 'Do older adults with early memory loss wish to be told if subsequently diagnosed with Alzheimer's disease?' *PSIGE Newsletter*, 99: 26–28.

Folstein, M.F., Folstein, S. and McHugh, P. (1975) 'Mini-mental state: a practical method for grading the cognitive state of patients for the clinician', *Journal of Psychiatric Research*, 12: 189–98.

Goldberg, D.P. and Hillier, V.F. (1979) 'A scaled version of the general health questionnaire', *Psychological Medicine*, 9: 139–45.

Graff, M.J.L., Vernooij-Dassen, M.J.M., Thijssen, M., Dekker, J., Hoefnagels, W.H.L. and OldeRikkert, M.G.M. (2006) 'Community based occupational therapy for patients with dementia and their caregivers', *British Medical Journal*, 333: 1196.

——(2007) 'Effects of Community Occupational Therapy on Quality of Life, Mood, and Health Status in Dementia Patients and their Caregivers: A Randomized Controlled Trial', *Journals of Gerontology Series A, Biological Sciences and Medical Sciences*, 62: 1002–9.

Kalbe, E., Kessler, J., Calabrese, P., Smith, R., Passmore, A.P., Brand, M. and Bullock, R. (2004) 'DemTect: a new sensitive cognitive screening test to support the diagnosis of mild cognitive impairment and early dementia', *International Journal of Geriatric Psychiatry*, 19: 136–43.

Laidlaw, K., Thompson, L.W., Dick-Siskin, L. and Gallagher-Thompson, D. (2003) *Cognitive Behaviour Therapy with Older People*, Chichester: Wiley.

Larner, A.J. (2007) 'DemTect: one year experience of a neuropsychological screening test for dementia', *Age and Ageing*, 36 (3): 326–27.

Lindesay, J., Marudkar, M., van Diepen, E. and Wilcock, G. (2002) 'The second Leicester survey of memory clinics in the British Isles', *International Journal of Geriatric Psychiatry*, 17: 41–47.

Lockwood, K.A., Alexopoulos, G.S. and van Gorp, W.G. (2002) 'Executive Dysfunction in Geriatric Depression', *American Journal of Psychiatry*, 159: 1119–26.

Malloy, D.M. and Standish, T.M. (1997) 'A guide to the standardised mini-mental state examination', *International Psychogeriatrics*, 9: 87–94.

Marzanski, M. (2000) 'Would you like to know what is wrong with you? On telling the truth to patients with dementia', *Journal of Medical Ethics*, 26: 108–13.

Mental Health and Older People Forum (2008) *A collective responsibility to act now on ageing and mental health. A consensus statement issued by key organisations integral to the support, care and treatment of mental health in later life*, London: Mental Health and Older People Forum.

Minshull, P. (2007) *Age equality: what does it mean for older people's mental health services?* North West Development Centre: Care Service Improvement Partnership.

Moniz-Cook, E., Gibson, G., Harrison, J. and Wilkinson, H. (2009) 'Timely psychosocial interventions in a memory clinic', in E.D. Moniz-Cook and J. Manthorpe (eds), *Early psychosocial interventions in dementia: Evidence-based practice*, London: Jessica Kingsley.

Moniz-Cook, E.D. and Manthorpe, J. (eds) (2009) *Early psychosocial interventions in dementia: Evidence-based practice*, London: Jessica Kingsley.

National Institute for Health and Clinical Excellence (2001) *Alzheimer's disease – donepezil, rivastigmine and galantamine for the treatment of Alzheimer's disease TA19*, London: National Institute for Health and Clinical Excellence. Available: www.nice.org.uk/TA19 (accessed 4 February 2010).

——(2007) *Alzheimer's disease – donepezil, galantamine, rivastigmine (review) and memantine for the treatment of Alzheimer's disease (amended) TA111*, London: National Institute for Health and Clinical Excellence. Available: www.nice.org.uk/TA111 (accessed 4 February 2010).

National Institute for Health and Clinical Excellence/Social Care Institute for Excellence (2006). *Dementia: supporting people with dementia and their carers in health and social care. NICE clinical practice guideline 42*, London: National Institute for Health and Clinical Excellence. Available: www.nice.org.uk/CG42 (accessed 4 February 2010).

Page, S., Hope, K., Bee, P. and Burns, A. (2008) 'Nurses making a diagnosis of dementia – a potential change in practice?' *International Journal of Geriatric Psychiatry*, 23: 27–33.

Phipps, A.J. and O'Brien, J.T. (2002) 'Memory Clinics and clinical governance – a UK perspective', *International Journal of Geriatric Psychiatry*, 17: 1128–32.

Potter, G.G., Kittinger, J.D., Wagner, H.R., Steffens, D.C. and Krishnan, K.R.R. (2004) 'Prefrontal neuropsychological predictors of treatment remission in later-life depression', *Neuropsychopharmacology*, 29: 2266–71.

Pratt, R. and Wilkinson, H. (2001) *'Tell me the truth' – The effect of being told the diagnosis of dementia from the perspective of the person with dementia*, London: Mental Health Foundation.

Quinn, C., Clare, L., Pearce, A. and van Dijkhuizen, M. (2008) 'The experience of providing care in the early stages of dementia. An interpretative phenomenological analysis', *Aging and Mental Health*, 12 (6): 769–78.

Roth, M., Huppert, F.A., Mountjoy, C.Q. and Tym, E. (1988) *CAMDEX-R: The Cambridge Examination for Mental Disorders in the Elderly – Revised*, Cambridge: Cambridge University Press.

Wechsler, D. (1997) *Wechsler Memory Scale – 3rd UK Edition (WMS-III UK)*, Oxford: Psychological Corporation/Pearson.

——(1999) *Wechsler Adult Intelligence Scale – 3rd UK Edition (WAIS-III UK)*, Oxford: Psychological Corporation/Pearson.

——D. (2001) *Wechsler Test of Adult Reading – UK Edition (WTAR UK)*, Oxford: Psychological Corporation/Pearson.

Wilson, B.A., Alderman, N., Burgess, P.W., Emslie, H. and Evans, J.J. (1996) *Behavioural Assessment of Dysexecutive Syndrome*, Oxford: Pearson.

Wright, N. and Lindesay, J. (1995) 'A survey of memory clinics in the British Isles', *International Journal of Geriatric Psychiatry*, 10: 379–85.

Yesavage, J.A., Brink, T.L., Lum, O., Huang, V., Adey, M.B> and Leirer, V.O. (1983) 'Development and validation of a geriatric depression screening scale: A preliminary report', *Journal of Psychiatric Research*, 17: 37–49.

Zigmond, A.S. and Snaith, R.P. (1983) 'The Hospital Anxiety and Depression Scale', *Acta Psychiatrica Scandinavica*, 67: 361–70.

8   The Croydon Memory Service

Using generic working to create efficiency, job satisfaction and satisfied customers

Rosalind Willis, Jenifer Chan, Issy Scriven, Vanessa Lawrence, David Matthews, Joanna Murray and Sube Banerjee

Key messages

- Memory clinics have been identified as key to delivering good quality early diagnosis and intervention.
- The Croydon Memory Service (CMS) operates a generic model of service delivery. The impact of generic working on staff and key stakeholders has yet to be evaluated within the literature.
- Generic working was found to create efficient working practices, a positive working environment and a supportive service for clients.
- The CMS model fostered teamwork and the professional identify of the different practitioners. Staff speculated on work stressors, but had not experienced negative aspects of generic working.
- General practitioners (GPs) valued the CMS policy of making and breaking the diagnosis of dementia to the older adult and their family. This facilitated open discussion on the illness.

Introduction

Memory clinics have been developing in the United Kingdom (UK) since the 1980s, and have been presented as an efficient way to identify cases of mild to moderate dementia and instigate and monitor drug treatment, as recommended by the *National Service Framework for Older People* (Department of Health 2001). Both nationally and internationally, memory clinics vary in their aims, scope and services provided (Lindesay *et al.* 2002, Dukes 2003), but they usually have the common aspects of assessing and diagnosing mild to moderate dementia. In England, the *National Dementia Strategy* suggests that memory clinics may form the core of new specialist services designed to deliver good quality early diagnosis and intervention (Department of Health 2009). A more complete review of memory clinic service provision can be found in the preceding chapter (Chapter 7), by Sue Watts and her colleagues.

The research setting

The Croydon Memory Service (CMS) is a form of memory clinic focused on the identification and treatment of people with mild to moderate dementia. It is a multi-disciplinary team, involving nursing, psychiatry, social work and psychology, and the team leader is a clinical psychologist. CMS has been operating since November 2002. A more detailed description of the service has been reported elsewhere (Banerjee *et al.* 2007). The treatments offered to those with mild to moderate dementia include the anti-dementia drugs (the acetylcholinesterase inhibitors), social interventions, and individual and group psychological therapies.

Generic working

CMS is a specialist secondary mental health service which is generic in terms of its model of service provision, further developing the 'Guy's model' (Collighan *et al.* 1993, Herzberg 1995, and see Chapter 6 in this book by Rahul (Tony) Rao and his colleagues for a more complete discussion on the 'Guy's model'). This means that any member of the team, regardless of professional background, can conduct the initial assessment. The generic model was adopted for the purposes of efficiency, to eliminate the logistical problem in the 'traditional' psychiatric service design where everybody needs to be seen by a doctor. This was intended to increase the capacity of the CMS to process cases and to reduce waiting times. Diagnoses and treatment and management plans are agreed at the weekly team meeting, with input from all disciplines. Any member of the team can order investigations, arrange for support services, hold followup meetings and otherwise manage cases, allowing for consistency of key worker throughout the assessment and treatment process.

Gehlhaar described some GPs who were 'suspicious' about multidisciplinary assessments (Gehlhaar 1988). However, Collighan *et al.* (1993) showed that the assessments made using the 'Guy's model' were as accurate as those made by expert research psychiatrists. Herzberg reported that with time and experience, GPs in North Southwark found the 'Guy's model' acceptable (Herzberg 1995).

Working in a generic team is associated with role blurring, which can lead to role ambiguity and stress (Burns 2001, Harries and Gilhooly 2003, Reeves and Summerfield Mann 2004). Working with older people, and also working with dementia (the two are not necessarily inextricable), have both been associated with stress (Banerjee 2001). It could therefore be expected that working at a service such as the CMS would lead to staff stress. The majority of models of employee health and job dissatisfaction focus upon stressors such as role conflict and role ambiguity (Bedeian and Armenakis 1981), poor fit between the person and the work environment (Kahn *et al.* 1964), and outcomes such as poor retention or burnout (Shirom 2003). Nelson and Simmons advocated examining the positive aspects of job satisfaction alongside the negative aspects leading to stress (Nelson and Simmons 2003).

Aim

While there are descriptions of specific generic teams in the literature, there has been no exploration of the effect working generically has on staff or stakeholders such as referrers, clients and family carers. Therefore, we completed a qualitative study to investigate further generic working. We used qualitative methods because of the low level of information available and because we wished to understand the experiences of three groups: CMS staff; GP referrers; and clients and carers.

Methods: participants

1   CMS staff
    A complete sample of CMS staff members was sought. Twelve staff members were asked to take part and all consented. The interviews were conducted between January and July 2004. These data remain both relevant and novel as the CMS continues to represent an innovative model of care and there is a continued absence of evidence within this field.

2   GPs
    The first 16 consecutive GPs who made referrals to the CMS were invited to participate; four declined, one had moved away, and one did not consent to being tape-recorded. A total of 10 GPs were therefore included in the analysis. The interviews took place between January and May 2004.

3   Clients and carers
    Purposive sampling was used to identify a group of clients and carers with a mix of demographic characteristics, and differing views about CMS. Forty people were approached for interview; sixteen clients and 15 carers consented and were interviewed. The interviews took place between March and August 2004. Recruitment ceased when theoretical saturation was reached, i.e. when no new themes emerged from data analysis.

Interviews

The interview guides were drawn up from the literature, refined on the basis of discussions with the project supervisors, and piloted upon non-involved clinical and research workers. The schedules were subject to iterative change; some questions were re-framed after the first few interviews, and some other questions were included that had emerged as important points in the early interviews. The CMS staff interviews focused on the experience of working in the service; the GP interviews focused on their expectations and experiences of making a referral to CMS; and the client and carer interviews focused on their experiences and evaluation of CMS.

   Local Research Ethics approval was obtained. Informed written consent was obtained, and confidentiality and the voluntary nature of the research were reinforced. The interviews lasted between 30 minutes and one hour. The interviews were semi-structured and took the form of a conversation framed around the interview guide, including prompts and queries to elicit more information or clarification. Interviews were conducted by three researchers (RW, JC, IS), two of whom had a dual role of clinician and researcher (JC, IS), while one was an independent researcher (RW). All staff interviews were conducted by the independent researcher. The client and carer interviews were conducted by RW and JC, who had not encountered the participants in the clinical setting. The researchers went to great lengths to emphasise their independence from CMS, and the confidential nature of the research. The person who interviewed the GPs (IS) did not have any other contact with the GPs.

Analysis

The interviews were tape recorded and transcribed. The three groups of interviews were analysed separately. The NVivo 2 (QSR 2002) qualitative data handling computer package was used in order to aid storage and coding of the interviews. Coding and analysis were conducted by the interviewers (RW, JC, IS). The interview transcripts were examined using Conventional Content Analysis (Hsieh and Shannon 2005). Open codes were drawn directly from the data. Coding frameworks were developed through discussion with other researchers not involved with this study but familiar with qualitative research. This ensured the coding decisions were trustworthy. The open codes of related meaning were condensed into higher order themes. Three themes related to generic working will be discussed in this chapter: 1 generic working equals efficiency and quality; 2 generic working leads to job satisfaction and satisfied customers; 3 negative aspects of generic working. These themes will now be expanded on below.

Results

Theme 1: generic working equals efficiency and quality.

Generic assessments and key work

Since all staff members have the skills necessary to assess clients, regardless of their clinical background, the progress of cases at CMS is more rapid and efficient than in traditional health care models. Further, because it is an integrated health and social care team, all staff members can also order specialist investigations and organise care packages for their cases:

> I think part of its strength is that each person does the same assessment and I think that although each person has a nominated role, they can work outside that role, so it's almost like everybody is on the same level. So it's not unusual for [the social worker] to be interviewing the person who has got the memory problems and the psychiatrist to be talking to the carer.
>
> (CMS staff 4)

The speed with which the CMS responded to referral impressed the GPs. Seven out of ten GPs told the interviewer that all of their clients had been seen quickly by the CMS, which was of great importance to the anxious clients and carers. GPs were also very impressed with the comprehensive assessment report they received on each case:

> This was an awful lot easier for me and it was certainly nicer for Mrs A and her relatives that it was fairly slick. Really I think, I think the Memory Service did pretty well.
>
> (GP10–17)

Fifteen of the 31 clients and carers who took part in the interviews spoke about the speed with which CMS had contacted them after the referral had been made. The majority were contacted by CMS within a month or less (13/15, 87 percent). All were happy with the speed of response to referral, and some remarked on how much better than ordinary NHS waiting times it was: 'I was staggered' (Carer 15).

Team decision making

All decisions about treatment and intervention are made through discussion and consensus at the multi-disciplinary team meetings. Each staff member has a voice in these meetings, even on issues outside of their own professional background:

The assessments are ... fed back to the team at the following team meeting and decisions are made regarding whether further investigation is required, whether neuropsych[ological] testing is required and once ... the entire assessment is completed ... decisions are made regarding appropriateness to treat in terms of medication or memory retraining. So decisions are very much team based. There's a flattened hierarchy and joint working.

(CMS staff 6)

Collaboration across disciplines

Key professions within health and social care are represented in the staff team, and there is an encouragement to turn to these specialists with queries about their particular field. This promotes skills building within each staff member as they apply new skills and knowledge to their own cases. It further adds to the efficient nature of generic working to have such a wide knowledge base easily available:

We are a fully integrated team of ... social services and various professionals from the NHS working in the same manner so that we all take responsibility for clients, we all key work clients in the same way but we have got the potential to call upon expert assessments or impressions from professionals with the team.

(CMS staff 3)

Does not blur professional boundaries

It could be expected that the variety of tasks conducted by each staff member within the generic team, regardless of professional background, might blur the boundaries between the different disciplines, yet this did not appear to be the case. Indeed, their own specialities were seen as valuable assets to the team:

It's a team work situation without staff losing their individual skills, their individual professional skills, it's the best of both worlds.

(CMS staff 5)

All staff familiar with all cases

The fact that every staff member is familiar with each of the cases adds to efficiency. This is the result of the group discussions about cases, both informally and at MDT meetings. Clients and carers are encouraged to ring CMS whenever they have a worry or a query and ask for their key worker. In the event that the key worker is unavailable, any other staff member is able to speak to the client or carer knowledgeably about their case. This is considered to be a strength in current CMS working:

One thing that has struck me about the team compared to other teams that I've worked in is the extent to which, if the client rings up and their key worker isn't there, almost anyone else in the team would be able to speak to them about whatever their problem is because they'll know their case and they will be able to kind of give some help.

(CMS staff 7)

One stop shop

Once the client has accessed CMS, they are in a one stop shop for all the services they will need for dementia care. CMS has efficient links with all the appropriate agencies involved in dementia care and arranges services on behalf of the clients, without the need for further referral and re-assessment in each case:

> It's an encompassing assessment and the fact that we are able to then provide much of the support that's necessary from under one roof. If it's something that we can't provide from the team it's ourselves who will access it from another department so that cuts out the client having to make 14 phone calls and not really knowing what they are asking for, so it's one point of delivery really.
>
> (CMS staff 4)

Clients and carers recognised the one stop shop aspect of CMS. Ten participants described CMS as a central point of access to all necessary services:

> It's the whole lot in one place rather than different groups in different places. It's like you get all, everybody you need in one place, so that's very helpful.
>
> (Carer 12)

The GPs also reflected that CMS appeared able to provide a seamless point of access to other services. This was described as an unusual and valuable ability, compared with the difficulty GPs themselves have had with trying to access external service involvement for their own clients:

> Once the diagnosis has been confirmed it opens up a lot of extra support that you with your team approach have a much easier access to than I do. I mean, I do have access to it but it's so much easier for it to be done all in one go rather than me referring to lots of different places.
>
> (GP14–18)

Theme 2: generic working leads to job satisfaction and satisfied customers

Challenging and exciting

Working at CMS was described as a very attractive role. Staff spoke about their reasons for applying to work at CMS. These included expectations of what the work would be like, a chance to advance their career, and a desire to work within the CMS model. Staff expected, and found, that the new style of work would be exciting and challenging:

> The group work has been quite hard but a really good challenge, it's been really sort of, been quite a buzz to get it right.
>
> (CMS staff 7)

Client contact

Staff expressed interest in working with people with dementia and their carers, as well as the ethnic and cultural demographic of Croydon. The generic assessment style also meant that all staff would have a great deal of client contact, which in a non-generic team would not necessarily be the case:

> I enjoy the, working with both the carer and the clients ... I enjoy the therapeutic contact with them both.
>
> (CMS staff 6)

Clients and carers valued the continuity of having a key worker from initial assessment throughout the treatment and management:

> It's reassuring. You can't, don't have to explain every time what you think, what's going on and so on.
>
> (Client 3)

Autonomy

The professional autonomy within the group setting was valued. Staff members were trusted to conduct assessments and make judgements about clients' and carers' needs. Further, if a staff member had any ideas about improvements which could be made, then there was a sense that these would be listened to by the senior staff:

> I had the freedom in that I was ... trusted ... enough to ... get on with it and I felt that if I had ideas on how things could be done differently or things that needed to be looked into, that they were actually listened to and that they were actually implemented.
>
> (CMS staff 5)

Feeling valued

The extent to which each staff member was made to feel that they were a valuable, essential and competent part of the team meant a great deal to the interviewees:

> Feeling valued, really feeling part of a team, not pretending to be part of a team, feeling that you are, that what you say does count and it doesn't matter what [level of seniority] you are.
>
> (CMS staff 9)

Chance to learn new skills

The expectation to learn new skills was perceived positively by the staff. They seemed to enjoy the challenge and appreciated the chance to develop new aspects of their professional abilities:

> I enjoy the fact that I have had the chance to do some, kind of go into research a bit, it was one of the areas that I didn't think I'd have much involvement with when I took this job and was one of the things that I was interested in.
>
> (CMS staff 2)

One of the new tasks the staff were required to carry out was delivering the diagnosis to the client and their carer. Traditionally, only a medic would be in this position. This was perceived as an important and powerful aspect of the role, if a slightly daunting one:

> Another new dimension of my work here is giving diagnoses because I have always been there, either, before this job, either encouraging GPs to refer for a diagnosis or picking up the pieces once the person is diagnosed, supporting and understanding, but here of course we have to go through the process of giving diagnoses.
>
> (CMS staff 1)

Four GPs reported that once CMS had named the diagnosis, the previously unmentionable word of dementia became usable:

> Quite often after they come back to us they're quite reassured. They have got oral diagnosis of dementia and it's suddenly discussable.
>
> (GP-2)

Faith in treatment model

The conviction that their work was benefiting clients and carers also enthused the staff and contributed to their continuing motivation and dedication to their work:

> Certainly I could see a change over the course of the [memory retraining] group which runs for six weeks. Kind of, her becoming much more relaxed, much less stressed and they seemed happier as a couple, more comfortable with each other and he gained a greater awareness of his memory difficulties.
>
> (CMS staff 7)

This faith is reinforced by the views expressed in the client and carer interviews. Eight of the people interviewed attended the memory retraining group, and all had positive things to say about it. Two of the people interviewed attended the carers' group, and said that it helped to address the emotional aspects of the caring role.

Theme 3: negative aspects of generic working

There were only two potential negative aspects of generic working mentioned in any of the interviews. Although CMS staff speculated about *potentially* negative aspects of working generically, there was currently no evidence of either.

Concern about the breadth of responsibility

A concern was raised by CMS staff that the work might be stressful, although no participant actually identified it as such. The novelty of the style of working was mentioned as a possible stressor for a new member of staff. Similarly, the breadth of the work staff members were expected to undertake outside their traditional professional background could be perceived as threatening at first. A specific stressor of working at CMS, raised by one member of staff, was the incurable nature of dementia. Finally, the increasing referral rate had a corresponding demand on the time of the key workers to carry out assessments:

> I also think that the way of working can lead to some pressure because it's an unre- mitting aspect of the work, the assessments don't stop, they are assessments that will need to go on week after week so it can be quite unremitting whereas traditionally that may not have been the case, that would have been the role of the psychiatrist to do the initial assessment but now we are all sharing that potential role.
>
> (CMS staff 3)

Concern that clients might prefer a medical key worker

There was a perception among three staff members that clients and carers could potentially react negatively to being seen by a generic staff member rather than a doctor or psychiatrist, but this had not yet been their experience:

> Well I would guess it could be perceived as a negative because we are working with a patient group in a generation who are maybe not as, I can't think of the word to use really, who maybe would prefer to actually just have a doctor see them in the clinic and a doctor make the diagnosis. I think that it might be a bit unsettling to people.
>
> (CMS staff 5)

The issue of the key worker not necessarily being a doctor did not seem to be a pro- blem to the clients and carers. None of them mentioned this issue at all. Similarly, GP referrers did not mention being unhappy with the initial assessment being carried out by non-medical staff.

Summary

Thus, the themes that emerged from the interviews focused on how CMS works and how this impacts upon staff, referrers, and clients and carers. The generic nature of the team gave rise to efficient working, which in turn resulted in high work satisfaction among CMS staff and produced benefits for GP referrers, clients and carers. There were two potential negative aspects raised about generic working. These positive and negative aspects of CMS team working are summarized in Table 8.1.

Discussion

The efficiencies arising from the CMS's generic style of working included: short wait- ing time between referral and assessment; maximising the numbers that can be seen; team decision-making; collaboration across disciplines without blurring professional boundaries; all staff being familiar with all cases; and a one stop shop for the complex needs of dementia care. The efficiency of the team was noted by GP referrers and also by clients and carers.

The issue of job stress was raised in the CMS staff interviews. The breadth of respon- sibilities each staff member faces, as well as the particular stresses of working with an incurable illness, were both highlighted as issues which could hypothetically be a cause

Table 8.1 The benefits of a generic team

Generic working equals ... Efficiency	And leads to ... Job satisfaction and satisfied customers	But potentially causes ...
• Generic assessments and key working • Team decision making • Collaboration across disciplines but does not blur professional boundaries • All staff familiar with all cases • One stop shop for assessments and treatments	• Exciting and challenging • Lots of client contact for all staff • Autonomy • Swift response to referral • Staff feel valued • Chance to learn new skills • Support for clients and carers • Full range of care for clients and carers • Faith in treatment model • Customer satisfaction	• Occupational stress? • Problems where generic keyworker is not a medic?

of job-related stress. However, none of the staff members considered themselves stressed by their work. Quite the contrary, the nature of the new team may have protected against potential stresses; in a similar way Herzberg wrote that the 'Guy's model' of working resulted in job satisfaction because staff felt that their skills and experience were valued by the team (Herzberg 1995). Further, the supportive nature of group decision-making may have protected against the stressful nature of the work.

As well as the aspects common to each role, each staff member also utilises their own professional discipline's skills, so there is less opportunity to lose a sense of one's own professional identity. There are suggestions from the occupational therapy literature that working generically causes a reduction in role clarity (Harries and Gilhooly 2003, Reeves and Summerfield Mann 2004), but this may have been minimised in the CMS by the fact that not all time is spent in generic working.

GPs agreed that the policy of CMS of communicating the diagnosis to both client and carer had great benefits for them, enabling them once the words had been said to engage in open discussion of treatment, management and future care. GPs appeared happy that the CMS made the diagnosis and broke that diagnosis to the person with dementia and their family carers for them. It seems likely that once the taboo words (dementia, or Alzheimer's disease) have been used by the 'experts', then this enables GPs to use the word too. Preliminary data from a memory clinic in Canada (Morgan *et al.* 2009) suggest that clients and families also appreciate receiving a diagnosis in this context.

Gehlhaar (1988) reported that GP referrers were uncomfortable with psychogeriatric assessments conducted by non-medical staff. Times have moved on in terms of generic working and there was no evidence of this in the current study. In fact, the GPs were impressed with the information and interventions they and their patients received and were not concerned that they were not provided directly by a doctor. This was mirrored by the finding that clients and carers were satisfied with the care provided and with not necessarily being assessed by a doctor.

The efficiency of the generic approach resulted in job satisfaction (because of challenging and exciting work), a high level of client contact, autonomy, the feeling of being valued, a chance to learn new skills, and faith in the treatment model. The positive aspects of the treatment were reinforced by the clients and carers. The consistency of having a key worker from the point of assessment onward, facilitated by the generic approach, was valued by clients and carers, as reported elsewhere (Willis *et al.* 2009). They described the benefits of not having to explain their situation anew each time they had contact with the service. The continuity was seen as reassurance, especially important for people coping with a distressing illness. This appears to be a marker of improved quality care.

One limitation of this study is that at the time of the research reported here the CMS was a relatively new team; it may be that the enthusiasm observed is a temporary phenomenon. New teams have been found to have a degree of optimism not present in established teams (Cook, Howe and Veal 2004, Kneafsey *et al.* 2004), and which has been described as a 'start-up effect' (Simpson and de Silva 2003). Another limitation is what might appear to be a relatively small number of respondents. However, this is a qualitative study and we used best quality methodology including continuing interviews to the point of data saturation. The fact that this is a study of a single service will affect the generalisability of the data and the themes generated, but this was intended as an evaluation of this particular model.

Even given these limitations this evaluation does present new data which support the development and use of models of generic working. The data suggest that such an approach can deliver good quality efficient services for people with dementia and their carers, which are acceptable to them and to the referring GPs.

References

Banerjee, S. (2001) 'Services for older adults', in G. Thornicroft and G. Szmukler (eds), *Textbook of Community Psychiatry*, Oxford: Oxford University Press.

Banerjee, S., Willis, R., Matthews, D., Contell, F., Chan, J. and Murray, J. (2007) 'Improving the quality of care for mild to moderate dementia: an evaluation of the Croydon Memory Service Model', *International Journal of Geriatric Psychiatry*, 22: 782–88.

Bedeian, A.G. and Armenakis, A.A. (1981) 'A path-analytic study of the consequences of role conflict and ambiguity', *Academy of Management Journal*, 24: 417–24.

Burns, T. (2001) 'Generic versus specialist mental health teams', in G. Thornicroft and G. Szmukler (eds), *Textbook of Community Psychiatry*, Oxford: Oxford University Press.

Collighan, G., Macdonald, A., Herzberg, J., Philpot, M. and Lindesay, J. (1993) 'An evaluation of the multidisciplinary approach to psychiatric diagnosis in elderly people', *British Medical Journal*, 306: 821–24.

Cook, S., Howe, A. and Veal, J. (2004) 'A different ball game altogether: Staff views on a primary mental healthcare service', *Primary Care Mental Health*, 2: 77–89.

Department of Health (2001) *National Service Framework for Older People*, London: Department of Health.

——(2009) *Living Well with Dementia: A National Dementia Strategy*, London: Department of Health.

Dukes, C. (2003) 'Memory clinics – current and future developments', *Dementia Bulletin*, November: 1–4.

Gehlhaar, E. (1988) 'Service evaluation in old age psychiatry: Using the general practitioner's view', *Psychiatric Bulletin*, 12: 428–30.

Harries, P.A. and Gilhooly, K. (2003) 'Generic and specialist occupational therapy casework in community mental health teams', *British Journal of Occupational Therapy*, 66: 101–9.

Herzberg, J. (1995) 'Can multidisciplinary teams carry out competent and safe psychogeriatric assessments in the community?' *International Journal of Geriatric Psychiatry*, 10: 173–77.

Hsieh, H.F. and Shannon, S.E. (2005) 'Three approaches to qualitative content analysis', *Qualitative Health Research*, 15: 1277–88.

Kahn, R.L., Wolfe, D.M., Quinn, R.P., Snoek, R.D. and Rosenthal, R. (1964) *Organisational stress: Studies in role conflict and ambiguity*, New York: John Wiley and Sons.

Kneafsey, R., Long, A., Reid, G. and Hulme, C. (2004) 'Learning and performing care management: Experiences of a newly formed interdisciplinary, assessment and rehabilitation team', *Learning in Health and Social Care*, 3: 129–40.

Lindesay, J., Marudkar, M., van Diepen, E. and Wilcock, G. (2002) 'The second Leicester survey of memory clinics in the British Isles', *International Journal of Geriatric Psychiatry*, 17: 41–47.

Morgan, D.G., Crossley, M., Kirk, A., D'Arcy, C., Stewart, N., Biem, J., Forbes, D., Harder, S., Basran, J., Bello-Haas, V.D. and McBain, L. (2009) 'Improving access to dementia care: development and evaluation of a rural and remote memory clinic', *Aging & Mental Health*, 13: 17–30.

Nelson, D.L. and Simmons, B.L. (2003) 'Health psychology and work stress: A more positive approach', in J.C. Quick and L.E. Tetrick (eds), *Handbook of Occupational Health Psychology*, Washington, DC: American Psychological Association.

QSR (2002) *NVivo 2*, Victoria, Australia: QSR International Pty Ltd.

Reeves, S. and Summerfield Mann, L. (2004) 'Overcoming problems with generic working for occupational therapists based in community mental health settings', *British Journal of Occupational Therapy*, 67: 265–68.

Shirom, A. (2003) 'Job related burnout: A review', in J.C. Quick and L.E. Tetrick (eds), *Handbook of Occupational Health Psychology*, Washington, DC: American Psychological Association.

Simpson, S. and de Silva, P. (2003) 'Multi-disciplinary team assessments: A method of improving the quality and accessibility of old age psychiatry services', *Psychiatric Bulletin*, 27: 346–48.

Willis, R., Chan, J., Murray, J., Matthews, D. and Banerjee, S. (2009) 'People with dementia and their family carers' satisfaction with a memory service: a qualitative evaluation generating quality indicators for dementia care', *Journal of Mental Health*, 18: 26–37.

9   Dementia
Complex case work

Karin Terri Smith and Lorna Mackenzie

Key messages

- The Newcastle Challenging Behaviour Team has a staff-centred and person-focused approach.
- Holistic assessment approach, including life story and experiences, physical and mental health.
- Conceptualizing the challenging behaviour, identifying the underlying need.
- Interventions – communication, approaches, consistency and continuity of care.
- Activity – providing the person with purposeful activity.

Introduction

The aim of this chapter is to demonstrate the use and efficacy of the Newcastle Challenging Behaviour Team's (NCBT) approach for residents in care homes whose behaviour has been labelled 'challenging'. The NCBT employs a staff-centred, person-focused approach that has been used over the last 10 years in 82 care facilities in the Newcastle area in the north-east of England. Most of the team's referrals are for people with dementia, but the NCBT also works with people with other mental health conditions, such as schizophrenia and/or depression. Our approach involves gathering specific information about the referred person's background and how he or she experiences the episode of behaviour that challenges (James and Stephenson 2007). Each care facility receives a 12-week intervention package (introduced later in the chapter) based around the 'problematic behaviour' which includes staff teaching and training. The approach builds upon Cohen-Mansfield's (2000) needs-led model which conceptualises the identified behaviour as the expression of an underlying need, e.g. as a drive to be free from pain, boredom, distress, fear, or an over-controlling environment. Understanding someone's behaviour in terms of this 'needs framework' enables staff to see the situation in a more positive light. It allows staff to empathise with the resident's situation and gives an opportunity to reflect upon what the resident might be feeling and what their own needs might be if they were placed in a similar situation. This approach places the person with dementia at the centre of the assessment and intervention process, requiring the carers (therapists, staff and families) to examine the person's 'problematic behaviour' in terms of both contextual features (history, health, cognitive status, environment, etc.) and its characteristics (frequency, severity, timing, etc.).

The team works primarily with the staff in the care home rather than the person who is presenting with the challenging behaviour, as it is this shift that is instrumental in bringing about and sustaining change. Team members work collaboratively with staff assisting to bring about a reduction in the behaviours.

The chapter will begin with a definition of dementia and challenging behaviour followed by a case study which will demonstrate the NCBT framework.

Definition of dementia and challenging behaviour

The term 'dementia' is used to describe the symptoms that occur when the brain is affected by specific diseases and conditions. Symptoms of dementia include loss of memory, confusion and problems with speech and understanding, and although there are many types of dementia, the most common are Alzheimer's disease, vascular dementia and Lewy Body dementia (Alzheimer's Society 2007). Other less common dementias include Frontal Lobe dementia, Parkinson's-related dementia and alcohol-related brain damage (Keady *et al.* 2009).

Dementia is generally progressive; therefore, the symptoms will tend to get worse. The trajectory will be different for each individual as regards how fast it progresses, and because each individual is unique, his/her experience of dementia will reflect this.

Typical symptoms of dementia include:

- Loss of memory – everyday examples would include: forgetting the last time he/she had a cup of tea or a meal; misplacing items; forgetting that a relative has just visited; forgetting appointments. The types of memory difficulties experienced by people with dementia are mostly language-based, i.e. declarative, and many of these language-based memories remain accessible if the person is provided with the correct cues. People with severe dementia can retain many of their memories, particularly action-based forms, i.e. procedural memories (James *et al.* 2007). Hence, if you place a piano in front of someone with dementia, he/she may not recall the name of the instrument, but be able to play it well.
- Poor concentration – due to this difficulty the person may be unable to sustain his/her attention for any prolonged period of time and also be easily distracted. Such problems may result in him/her being unable to read a newspaper, follow a television programme or maintain a conversation.
- Disorientation – the person might become confused about where he/she is, or where others are. He/she may even experience a time shift, being uncertain or incorrect about the date. Sometimes the person may not recognize his/her current home and may wish to return to a home he/she lived in previously.
- Poor insight – he/she may no longer be able to think through things in a balanced manner. For example, he/she may incorrectly think he/she is able to attend to his/her own hygiene needs or to dress himself/herself. Another example is a failure to appreciate that certain behaviours he/she is displaying are unacceptable, for instance excessive swearing.
- Confabulation – because of memory problems the person may have gaps in his/her recall, which may lead him/her to guess what happened during these times. This 'filling-in' is termed confabulation. Thus the person may appear to speak coherently, but later one may find aspects of the story were fabricated.
- Word finding difficulties – language problems are common in people with dementia and the difficulties may be at the level of production or comprehension, or both.

The examples listed above have focused on the cognitive deficits experienced by individuals. Clearly, the difficulties experienced by a person with dementia increase as one compounds the situation by adding to the mix the typical physical, physiological and sociological challenges associated with ageing. Figure 9.1 attempts to capture the key 'problematic features' experienced in dementia, particularly relating to those living in care. It is our team's belief that the issues outlined in this wheel, and residents' attempts to deal with them, lie behind a lot of the major 'behaviours that challenge' that are seen in care homes. For example, take a man who thinks he is in his 20s suddenly

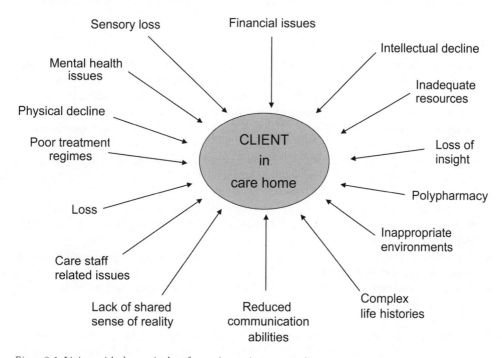

Figure 9.1 Living with dementia: key factors impacting on our client group.

Table 9.1 List of challenging behaviours

Aggressive behaviours: physical and verbal	Non-aggressive behaviours
• Kicking	• Wandering/restlessness
• Punching/slapping	• Repetitive behaviour, e.g. saying a phrase or word,
• Pushing or tugging	opening and closing a drawer
• Scratching	• Irritability/lability
• Biting/nipping	• Anxiety/attention seeking
• Threatening, e.g. waving a stick	• Disinhibited behaviour, e.g. sexual, stripping,
• Shouting	insensitive/hurtful comments
• Screaming	• Communication difficulties
• Weeping/sobbing	• Depression/apathy
• Bullying	• Hallucinations/delusions
• Swearing	• Sleeping disturbances
	• Appetite, e.g. over-/under-eating

finding himself being undressed by a young carer in his own bedroom. Such a situation may lead to an action subsequently labelled as 'sexual disinhibition'. Another example might be a recently widowed resident with word-finding difficulties and arthritis, communicating her need for comfort and relief from pain via 'shouting' or 'trailing'.

A list of commonly described 'behaviours that challenge' is provided in Table 9.1. It is vital not to view them as diagnostic categories because the label 'challenging' is only relevant to the context in which they are performed. Thus two different sets of care staff can often view the same behaviour differently, with only one group labelling the resident's actions as a challenging behaviour. Thus the items listed in Table 9.1 are really constructs, and their status as challenging will depend to an extent on the 'eye of the beholder'.

Prevalence and demographics

In 2006 the Alzheimer's Society commissioned the London School of Economics and the Institute of Psychiatry, King's College London to produce a report on dementia in the United Kingdom (UK). The research team was commissioned to provide the most up-to-date evaluation of the numbers of people with dementia in the UK and projections on numbers of people in the future (Alzheimer's Society 2007). As these demographic data revealed, the prevalence of both young-onset and late-onset dementia increases with age, doubling with every five-year increase across much of the age range. Moreover, the Alzheimer's Society (2007) report also indicated that:

- The prevalence of young-onset dementia (under 65 years old) was seen to be higher in men than in woman for those aged 50 – 65, while late-onset dementia was considered to be marginally more prevalent in women than in men.
- Alzheimer's disease was considered to be the dominant subtype, particularly among older people, and in women.
- The report estimates that there are 11,392 people from black and minority ethnic groups with dementia.

With respect to challenging behaviour, the prevalence rates are over 90 percent during the later stages of the illness (Ballard 2005). The impact of the behaviours can be marked, because they are associated with breakdown of care at home, institutionalisation, increased hospital admissions, transfer amongst care settings and increased costs (Moniz-Cook, Woods and Gardiner 2000).

Key policy drivers

The psychological approach used by the NCBT is in keeping with government health and social service policies. It is wholly consistent with the *National Dementia Strategy* for England (Department of Health 2009), particularly in relation to objectives 11 (living well with dementia in care homes) and 13 (developing an effective workforce). The Strategy sets out a vision for providing people who have dementia, and their carers, choice in the sorts of care they receive and also a viable alternative to tranquilising medications, as this quotation reveals:

> In this [current] system the quality of mental health care for residents in care homes could be improved by: ... the formulation and deployment of non-pharmacological

strategies for behavioural disorders in dementia, so avoiding the initiation of anti-psychotic medication; a rapid response to problems as they occur within homes; and assessments of the residential care provided and the potential for improvement – to create a more therapeutic environment.

(Department of Health 2009: 73)

The rallying call for the use of non-pharmacological alternatives to current medication regimens is echoed in numerous other documents. For example, *Always a Last Resort*, prepared by an All Party Parliamentary Group (APPG), recommended that psychological interventions and staff training in dementia care should be prioritised (All Party Parliamentary Group 2009). The National Institute for Health and Clinical Excellence/Social Care Institute for Excellence (2006) guideline *Dementia: supporting people with dementia and their carers in health and social care* (*NICE clinical practice guideline 42*) also recommends the use of specific behaviour analysis conducted by trained professionals.

Despite such endorsements, it is clear that the most commonly used treatment for problematic behaviours is medication. Indeed, research has highlighted that a high proportion of care home residents with dementia receive treatment for challenging behaviour with major anti-psychotics (James, Wood-Mitchell and Waterworth 2006). For example, prior to the introduction of guidelines in 1987 in the USA, it was estimated that 43 percent–55 percent of residents were receiving anti-psychotics. In recent surveys conducted on the use of anti-psychotics in nursing homes in the UK, it was found that between 24 percent (McGrath and Jackson 1996) and 36 percent (Dempsey and Moore 2005) of residents were prescribed such medication. In residential homes, the rate of prescribing was also high, at 29 percent (Dempsey and Moore 2005): see Table 9.2.

These rates are particularly worrying owing to the modest level of evidence for the efficacy of this medication (Sink, Holden and Yaffe 2004). The researchers also noted that work needed to be conducted on the side-effects, as the use of these drugs has been associated with an increased risk of falls, drowsiness, Parkinsonism, akathisia, tardive dyskinesias, neuroleptic sensitivity reactions and accelerated cognitive decline (McShane *et al.* 1997). Furthermore, there are specific concerns about the cardiotoxicity of thioridazine, and the increased risk of cerebro-vascular events in patients taking this group of drugs.

Applying principles

The NCBT was developed because of a gap in the existing clinical services, which meant that some of the most complex people in our communities were not receiving adequate care. Traditionally, the private sector care homes had proven difficult places to work into, because they had not previously received sustained attention from NHS therapists. Thus they had become rather wary of input when it was offered, preferring

Table 9.2 Use of psychotropic medication in non-EMI (nursing and residential) care homes in the UK

Area and study	Anti-psychotics	Benzodiazepines	Antidepressants
South of England (MacDonald *et al.* 2002)	15%	24%	25%
Yorkshire (Dempsey and Moore 2005)	31%	21%	22%

medication to therapy, and the commitments the latter involved. This, in turn, had made NHS therapists reluctant to engage with such environments due to the poor reception that was often received. In order to break this negative cycle, the NCBT was established. Initially, it comprised a psychologist and a nurse, and was piloted for two years. The remit of this team was mainly clinical, but it was quickly recognised that teaching and supervision would need to play important roles in the work of the team. As the team grew, the NCBT became more involved in conducting action-based research, and to date it has more than 70 publications to its name (see for example, Wood-Mitchell *et al.* 2008, Smith, Milburn and Mackenzie 2008, and Mackenzie, Wood-Mitchell and James 2007).

Currently the team consists of five mental health nurses. It is managed by a psychologist and receives sessional input from a psychiatrist. Over the last decade 867 people have received the above approach; currently the NCBT sees approximately 200 residents per year. Empirical evaluation of the work has demonstrated its efficacy (Wood-Mitchell *et al.* 2007). In recent years the approach has been adopted by, and informed the development of, other services in the UK (Northern Ireland, London, Aberdeen, Sheffield, Southampton, etc.). We believe the reason for its success is to do with its values and that it empowers all of those involved in dealing with the problematic behaviour (i.e. the resident, staff, family, care home manager). This systemic stance helps to ensure that the formulation-led care plans are initiated and adhered to appropriately.

To illustrate how behaviour that challenges can be addressed using the NCBT approach, a case study is presented: Rebecca. It is relevant to note that the NCBT recognises the important role medication has to play in the care of people with dementia, but it is only one element of an holistic approach.

Case study

Rebecca, aged 103, diagnosed with Alzheimer's disease, was referred to the NCBT following a request from the care home staff. Staff had been concerned about her aggression particularly towards other residents. On one occasion she shut a door in the face of a fellow resident and on another scratched the arm of a member of staff. The home manager had asked the general practitioner (GP) to give her a physical examination to rule out any physical causes for the behaviour; none were found.

Once referred to the NCBT, the standard pathway of care was initiated as outlined in Table 9.3. All residents accepted by the team receive this 12-week package of care delivered by an experienced therapist.

The steps outlined in Table 9.3 are now discussed below under the headings of Assessment, Information Sharing Sessions and Interventions, and Formulation and Care Planning.

Assessment

Discussions with staff: On the first visit to the home by the NCBT therapist, staff stated that the inappropriate behaviour displayed by Rebecca usually occurred around personal care activities. They felt it important to note that over the last couple of years, this proud and independent woman had become more dependent on the staff to meet her hygiene needs. In addition, they reported that she had recently begun to walk up and down the corridor shouting, 'Help me; please help me'. However, when asked

Table 9.3 Pathway of Newcastle Challenging Behaviour Team

Structure and timing	Action: what a team member should do
Week 1: initial input	• Receive referral • Request information (hospital case notes) and contact other professionals who have been involved previously • Complete initial documentation • Ensure physical checks have been done • Contact home to make initial appointment and check difficulties have not been resolved • Inform referrer and GP
Week 2: visit to the care facility	• Speak to manager/care staff, obtaining perceptions • Explain nature of service, including commitment and team's expectations of home • Speak to, or see, client • Complete baseline assessment • Go through notes held in care home • Discuss observation charts with staff and leave them in care facility • Conduct a risk assessment • Check with home that family/advocates are aware of team's involvement
Week 3: collate and review information	• Collect information and charts from home • Review need for additional information • Meet with family and obtain background information • Specify and clarify nature of difficulties • Arrange feedback and problem solving session with staff (i.e. formulation session)
Weeks 4–5: care staff formulation sessions	• Feedback information obtained • Provide appropriate educational material • Encourage staff participation • Help identify patterns in behaviour and staff responses • Determine potential triggers • Collaboratively devise SMART interventions • Arrange further interventions (night staff, etc.)
Week 6: post session	• Provide home with typed summary sheet, and related interventions • Ask home to complete circulation sheet, which checks that staff have i) read, and ii) understood material • Inform referrer and GP of progress
Week 7: follow-up	• Review staff's perception of client's difficulties • If necessary, reformulate
Weeks 8–11	• Regular visits supporting staff and tweaking interventions
Week 12: discharge	• Discharge with three months' direct re-referral access to service

what was wrong, she would say: 'There is nothing wrong'. Below is a typical report of a 'problematic' behaviour:

> When Rebecca is incontinent, she asks to be taken to the toilet to get washed and changed. However, as soon as she is in the bathroom she attempts to scratch and kick.

Discussions with Rebecca: She said that she has no complaints at all. When asked how she was, she replied: 'I'm fine, the staff here are nice'. Of note, during the conversation her memory difficulties and attentional problems became obvious. It was also evident that she lacked insight into the problems being caused by her behaviours and shouting. The discussions with Rebecca were supplemented with observations of her interactions with others (fellow residents and staff) in order to help in getting a clearer assessment of her difficulties.

During this visit an attempt was also made to complete a Mini-mental State Examination (MMSE) (Folstein, Folstein and McHugh 1975). Whilst attempting to complete the first section of the MMSE on orientation, Rebecca was aware that she could not answer the questions and became quite distressed. She held her head in her hands and stated: 'I should know this, why don't I know this, what is wrong with me?' The therapist thought that nothing could be gained by continuing and did not want to cause her any further distress and therefore abandoned the psychometric assessment.

At the initial interview Rebecca's key worker was asked to complete the Neuropsychiatric Inventory with caregiver distress (NPI-D; Cummings *et al*. 1994) as a baseline assessment. This is a scale which evaluates a range of behavioural disturbances; 12 areas are covered. It is scored from 1 to 144, with severity and frequency both assessed. The scale has well-established validity and reliability criteria (Cummings *et al*. 1994). The NPI-D version also includes a measure of carer distress, using a scale of 0–5 ('not at all' to 'severely distressed') for each behavioural area; this yields a score of 0 to 60. On the NPI-D Rebecca achieved high scores of 72 and 30 for the behavioural disturbance and carer distress, respectively.

Information gathering: The therapist's role during this stage was mainly to engage in a fact finding process in relation to both her past (biography, health status, etc.) and the present difficulties. Thus information about Rebecca was also obtained from case notes held in the care home and medical notes held at the hospital. She also gave permission for an examination of her GP notes. Further information was obtained from her friends who visited.

Significantly, the care notes in the home had very little information about Rebecca's background. They stated that she had been born in South Africa and that she played the cello professionally. Fortunately, her friend was a good source of information and she was asked to complete a Personal Profile form (see Table 9.4). This form is usually completed with a family member (a summary of the helpful information provided by the friend is given below).

Table 9.4 Personal profile: completed with family and/or friends; examples of questions asked

Personal details	*Personality*
• Where was he/she born and where did he/she grow up?	• Was the person pleasant or grumpy, introvert or extrovert, easy going or impatient, sociable or a loner, etc.?
• Parents', siblings' names	• Hobbies and interests
• School days and achievements	• Likes and dislikes (food, music, television, etc.)
• Lifetime experiences – good or bad	• Biggest achievement
• Religion/spiritual needs – customs, celebrations	• Proudest moment
• Important people in his/her life	• What would embarrass him/her
• Working life history	• What would upset him/her
• Any physical problems	• Saddest memories
• Any mental health problems	• Happiest memories

Summary of information obtained from Rebecca's friend:

- Rebecca was born in 1905 in South Africa. Rebecca's father was an electrical engineer who worked for a shipping company. Rebecca often spoke of her father with great respect and admiration. Rebecca's mother came from York. She worked as a secretary in London before she was married. She died in 1926. Rebecca's father was just too old to be drafted into the First World War. He died in his 100th year.
- The family returned to Tyneside when Rebecca was five. The journey home by ship, calling in at ports, remains one of Rebecca's enduring memories. The ship's captain was very kindly to children.
- Later she became a schoolmistress in Durham, teaching music. She also played in the Northern Philharmonic Orchestra, and enjoyed church music. For many years she shared a flat with Susan, but eventually Susan got married.
- Rebecca's family were Protestants. Importantly, she finds the iconography of traditional Christianity upsetting – she does not like pictures of Jesus on the cross.
- Rebecca used to be a whizz at Scrabble and still likes word searches. I did a jigsaw with her the other day and, after a slow start, she enjoyed it.
- Rebecca can be very bossy – she still thinks she is a school teacher!
- When Rebecca was on the first floor of this care facility, the chestnut tree outside her window gave her enormous pleasure. She would sit and look at it for hours, watching the leaves moving in the wind, the sunlight on the leaves, the flowers opening up in spring. Now she is on the top floor, there isn't much to see out of the window. She also likes 'people-watching' – watching the staff and other residents come and go without necessarily being close to them or interacting with them.

The therapist also spent time in the home observing Rebecca, and important information was obtained, using ABC behaviour charts, which identified the Antecedents of the Behaviour and the Consequences. For example, on one occasion, she spent most of the afternoon walking up and down the corridor repeating 'Please, please help me, please'. Initially it was a whisper, but gradually it got louder and louder until she was shouting. When asked what was wrong, Rebecca seemed surprised by the question then replied, 'I'm OK, why are you asking?' When the therapist said: 'You are saying please, please help me', she replied with a wave of her hand, 'Oh just ignore me. It's just a habit!'.

Once the therapist had collated the various pieces of information and devised the presentation format, an Information Sharing Session (ISS) was organized. This is a meeting that brings all the data together and presents them to the staff, giving the staff ownership of the work. At the end of this session a series of interventions is developed by the staff with the assistance of the therapist. The ISS is described in more detail below.

Information sharing session and interventions

The ISS is a 40- to 60-minute meeting co-ordinated by the therapist and is held at the care home. As many of the staff as possible are asked to attend, and usually around four or five staff attend each session. Often the sessions have to be repeated to ensure consistency and continuity with respect to the treatment plans developed from the meeting.

In the ISS, all the background information collected is presented and put together with the data from the ABC charts. During the session, the therapist helps the staff to make links and reflect on the behaviours in relation to the resident's needs. Once the assessment details have been discussed, a set of interventions is developed by the care staff with the assistance of the therapist.

In the case of Rebecca it became evident that up until this point the staff had very little knowledge and awareness of her background. After the data presentation, the following issues were particular foci of attention by the staff and therapist during the ISS.

Rebecca is:

- A very private and reserved lady. She was horrified if a male had to attend to her personal care needs because she was not used to having males around.
- A very intelligent, competent lady. Up until now she had always been in control of her life. She is particularly strong willed and single minded.
- A perfectionist and therefore doesn't like others saying she is unable to do things for herself.
- A spiritual person. She regularly attended Quaker meetings along with Christian Scientist meetings until recently.
- A single woman. She has never been married, never lived with anyone apart from her friend, who lived with her for 12 years. However, even then the friend had lived by Rebecca's rules.
- A single-minded individual. If she made a decision, she'd stick by it.
- A physically and mentally active lady. She was now frustrated with her circumstances, especially when finding it difficult to express herself.
- A 'bossy' person. She was an 'old style' school teacher.
- A lover of music. She loved classical music.
- An anxious individual. She was prone to anxiety when confused or unsure of what was expected of her.

Having discussed the above issues in some detail, a set of interventions and approaches were developed by the staff. It is relevant to note that the therapist played a major role in ensuring that the goals were realistic and feasible. Indeed, for each intervention the therapist is routinely instructed to employ the SMART criteria (Specific, Measurable, Appropriate, Realistic, Targeted), with respect to the goal-setting (Fossey and James 2008).

In the present case, two main groups of interventions were devised: the first to reduce her agitation around personal care activities, and the second to relieve her boredom. Indeed, in relation to the latter, it was hypothesised that her cries were due to lack of stimulation and boredom.

Formulation and care planning

Following the ISS a formulation framework was produced (see Figure 9.2). Much of the information in Figure 9.2 had already been presented to the staff in the ISS via a flip chart. This flip chart information had helped to generate discussion and assisted the staff to achieve a greater level of understanding regarding Rebecca's behaviour. However, in the next stage, the information discussed must be condensed and written up in the form of a single A4 sheet of paper, i.e. the formulation.

The experience of the NCBT suggests that supplying staff with an overly comprehensive formulation presented on multiple sheets is both off-putting and less likely to be read. In contrast, it has been found that a single formulation sheet, with a brief care plan attached, provides the most effective treatment strategy. Typically, the care plans

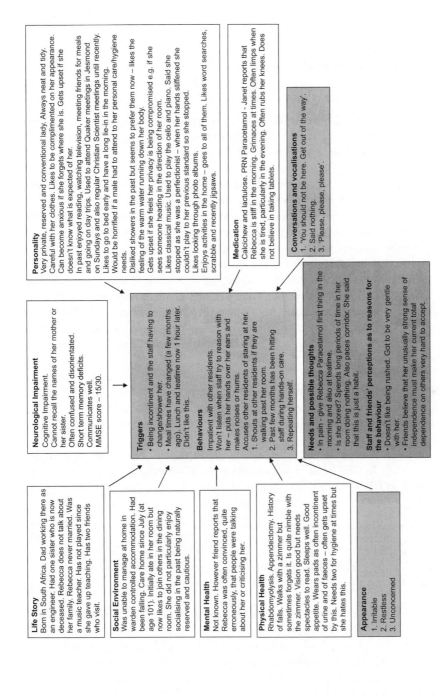

Life Story
Born in South Africa. Dad working there as an engineer. Had one sister who is now deceased. Rebecca does not talk about her family. Rebecca never married. Was a music teacher. Has not played since she gave up teaching. Has two friends who visit.

Social Environment
Was unable to manage at home in warden controlled accommodation. Had been falling. Care home since July (at age 101). Initially ate in her room but now likes to join others in the dining room. She did not particularly enjoy socialising in the past being naturally reserved and cautious.

Mental Health
Not known. However friend reports that Rebecca was often convinced, quite erroneously, that people were talking about her or criticising her.

Physical Health
Rhabdomyolysis. Appendectomy. History of falls. Walks with a zimmer but sometimes forgets it. Is quite nimble with the zimmer. Vision good but needs spectacles to read. Sleeps well. Good appetite. Wears pads as often incontinent of urine and of faeces – often gets upset by this. Needs two for hygiene at times but she hates this.

Appearance
1. Irritable
2. Restless
3. Unconcerned

Neurological Impairment
Cognitive Impairment.
Cannot recall the names of her mother or her sister.
Often confused and disorientated.
Short term memory deficits.
Communicates well.
MMSE score – 15/30.

Personality
Very private, reserved and conventional lady. Always neat and tidy. Careful with her clothes. Likes to be complimented on her appearance. Can become anxious if she forgets where she is. Gets upset if she doesn't know what is expected of her.
In past enjoyed reading, watching television, meeting friends for meals and going on day trips. Used to attend Quaker meetings in Jesmond on Sundays and also regular Christian Scientist meetings until recently. Likes to go to bed early and have a long lie-in in the morning.
Would be horrified if a male had to attend to her personal care/hygiene needs.
Disliked showers in the past but seems to prefer them now – likes the feeling of the warm water running down her body.
Gets upset if she feels her privacy is being compromised e.g. if she sees someone heading in the direction of her room.
Likes classical music. Used to play the cello and piano. Said she stopped as she was a perfectionist – when her hands stiffened she couldn't play to her previous standard so she stopped.
Likes looking through photo albums.
Enjoys activities in the home – goes to all of them. Likes word searches, scrabble and recently jigsaws.

Medication
Calcichew and lactulose. PRN Paracetamol - Janet reports that Rebecca is stiff in the morning. Grimaces at times. Often limps when she is tired, particularly in the evening. Often rubs her knees. Does not believe in taking tablets.

Conversations and vocalisations
1. 'You should not be here. Get out of the way'.
2. Said nothing.
3. 'Please, please, please'.

Triggers
• Being incontinent and the staff having to change/shower her.
• Meal times have changed (a few months ago). Lunch and teatime now 1 hour later. Didn't like this.

Behaviours
Impatient with other residents.
Won't listen when staff try to reason with her – puts her hands over her ears and makes noises or hums.
Accuses other residents of staring at her.
1. Shouts at other residents if they are walking past her room.
2. Past few months has been hitting staff during hands-on care.
3. Repeating herself.

Needs and possible thoughts
• In pain – give Rebecca Paracetamol first thing in the morning and also at teatime.
• Is she bored? Spends long periods of time in her room doing nothing. Also paces corridor. She said that this is just a habit.

Staff and friends' perceptions as to reasons for the behaviour
• Doesn't like being rushed. Got to be very gentle with her.
• Friends believe that her unusually strong sense of independence must make her current total dependence on others very hard to accept.

Figure 9.2 Rebecca: case formulation

are written summaries of the interventions derived from the ISS meetings. A summary of some of the care planning from Rebecca's case is given below. Note that the text has been written in a practical manner, and specific ideas have been attributed to staff. The information gathered from the assessment phase as well as the background information supplied by her friends is presented in Figure 9.2.

Summary – material for Rebecca's care plan

1 A few of the interventions suggested to assist with 'hands-on' care

Staff believe that the reason Rebecca becomes aggressive during assistance with personal care activities is because she is ashamed. Here are some tips suggested by the care workers Janet, Morag and Polly to try to reduce her embarrassment:

- If you notice she has been incontinent try saying: 'I think you've sat on something really dirty/really messy. Can I help get you clean and comfortable?'
- If you think Rebecca has been incontinent, staff have found it helpful to say to her 'Can I just check your pad?', rather than tell her she is wet or dirty. Staff also suggest that you try to be discreet when you are taking the pad off or putting it on. Morag says that she tries to take it off and slip a clean one on without Rebecca seeing it.
- Polly says that if Rebecca thinks there is a purpose to what you are asking her to do she will let you do it. Hence, when washing her breasts, one might say: 'Can I just check underneath to make sure they are not getting sore?' Try and give her a purpose for all aspects of personal care. For example, when Rebecca has been incontinent, try saying: 'Can I just take you to the toilet to check your bottom is not getting red and sore?'.
- Sometimes she goes to the toilet herself. Would regular prompting help? For example, one could say: 'I'm just going past the toilet, do you want to come with me?'.
- Be aware that Rebecca will tap her tummy when she needs the toilet.
- Also be aware that Rebecca is more agitated if she has a urinary tract infection or is constipated.
- Rebecca does not like to be disturbed when she is in the toilet. She worries that someone will walk in. She hates it when anyone knocks on the door. Try putting up a DO NOT DISTURB sign on the door when you take her.

2 A few of the interventions to relieve her agitation

If you notice Rebecca becoming agitated, sit her where she can see out of the window. Janet, Morag and Polly agreed that the dining room was the best place. Put a cushion behind her back and on the chair to make it more comfortable, otherwise she will not sit for long.

Rebecca enjoys nature; see Hazel's descriptions about the colours of the trees and so on. As a result, Polly suggested taking her to the garden centre. One may see if Rebecca wanted to choose some plants, bulbs or flowers that she could grow in her room (seasonal plants, e.g. daffodils, hyacinths for the spring, or cyclamen, poinsettia in the winter). Morag suggested a brightly coloured watering can so that Rebecca could tend the plants. Janet also suggested that the activities co-ordinator, Timothy, may be able to organise an activity with a gardening theme, for example painting plant pots.

3 A few of the interventions to relieve her boredom

Rebecca likes to watch some programmes on television: *The Weakest Link*; *Songs of Praise*; cookery programmes; nature programmes; *The Proms* or anything to do with the Royal Albert Hall. Rebecca may also enjoy looking through some books of Royalty or cookery books. If you look through her photograph album with her, the photographs seem to cue memories of her past. Other comments from the staff regarding enjoyable activities included:

- Rebecca enjoyed doing the jigsaw that her friend Hazel brought in.
- Talk to her about her life. She likes to talk about South Africa or the trip home when she was a girl. Also talk to her about her relatives who went to Australia or her sister's trip to Australia.
- Rebecca likes to watch other people. She may not want to join in with the activity, but she might enjoy 'people-watching'.
- It is important to be sensitive about the activities Rebecca is encouraged to do. Hazel gave an example: One day Timothy asked Rebecca to play bingo, but she declined immediately. Timothy was troubled by the strength of her reaction, and reckons it may have something to do with Rebecca's puritan background. She may class bingo as a form of gambling. Timothy was certainly right not to push the matter.
- Rebecca always enjoys looking through her photo album.
- Rebecca always enjoys the Jacqueline du Pré (cellist) DVD that Hazel brought in. Try using that if you have got time to sit down with her, or if another resident can sit with her.

Follow-up and outcome

After the intervention has been given to the staff, the remaining visits to the home by the NCBT staff are follow-up sessions. These are supportive visits designed to maintain consistency and provide encouragement. They are frequently not pre-arranged, and may only last for 15 minutes or so. For some residents the follow-up work may find that the formulation may require changing (or adding to), or the interventions tweaking. This was not the situation with Rebecca's case because she responded very well to the changes in attitudes and behaviour of the staff.

After a total of 12 weeks' input, Rebecca was discharged. At the final session a discharge interview took place. Her key worker was asked to complete the NPI-D again. Her scores on discharge showed a marked reduction, with a behavioural disturbance score of 11 and a caregiver distress score of 10.

Discussion and conclusion

There is limited evaluation of the impact of community teams working into care homes, with relatively few exceptions (Bullock 2002, James *et al.* 2006). This chapter has presented the work of the NCBT in Newcastle-upon-Tyne, UK, which provides input primarily into care settings. It aims to reduce challenging behaviour within private-sector homes and prevent, where appropriate, transfers and hospital admissions. The team uses a formulation model (James *et al.* 2006, James and Stephenson 2007) in order to develop targeted bio-psychosocial approaches. It works to minimise pharmacological

Table 9.5 Audit of Newcastle Challenging Behaviour Team – 2008/09

Feature	Number	Comments
Number of residents referred	170	
Number of residents referred who were subsequently admitted to a hospital ward	14	43% of the residents going into hospital were on the waiting list and had not yet been seen by team
Number of referred patients transferred to another care setting	9	The transfer was facilitated by NCBT, and often due to changes required to meet the resident's emerging needs (e.g. moving from a residential to nursing care setting)
Spontaneous recovery	41	A number of the residents who responded did not require the full formulation approach, but responded to use of pain relief, or monitoring, or simple advice from an NCBT member
Mean reduction NPI behaviour (pre – post score)	17.92	
Mean reduction carer distress	5.85	

use and also trials psychosocial approaches before psychotropic medication, in line with current national guidelines (Howard *et al*. 2001, Department of Health 2009). Where psychotropic approaches are felt to be required (e.g. psychosis, depression), the formulation assists with the tailoring of the approach to meet the needs of the individual (Gill *et al*. 2005).

An audit of the service (Wood-Mitchell *et al*. 2007) revealed the team to be effective on a number of levels. For example, there was a significant reduction in the pre- and post-NPI-D scores in terms of frequency and severity of behaviour, and caregiver distress. Additionally, only 5 percent of the referrals seen by the NCBT were admitted to a hospital ward, and only 9 percent transferred to another care setting. Taken together, these findings suggest that the team's approach is an effective method of dealing with 'behaviours that challenge' and staff distress. A more recent assessment revealed a similar profile as outlined in Table 9.5.

While examination of the data in Table 9.5 is reassuring, the evidence for the value of our work comes from observing the changes taking place within the care settings. The members of the NCBT attribute much of this to the use of the formulation-led model that seeks to identify residents' 'needs'. Indeed, it is evident that through this approach staff usually become motivated to learn more about the person and the causes of the problem behaviour. Thus, this method can be seen as a re-personalisation process. This is the reverse of Kitwood's (1997) notion of depersonalisation, whereby residents often lost their sense of identities due to staff not knowing, or not having regard for, residents' individual interests or personal histories. The re-personalisation process was clearly evident in the case of Rebecca, as it became clear early on that staff knew little about her.

References

All Party Parliamentary Group (2009) *Always a last resort: Inquiry into the prescription of antipsychotic drugs to people with dementia living in care homes*, London: Alzheimer's Society.

Alzheimer's Society (2007) *Dementia UK: A report into the prevalence and cost of Dementia, prepared by the Personal Social Services Research Unit (PSSRU) at the London School of Economics and the Institute of Psychiatry at King's College London for the Alzheimer's Society*, London: Alzheimer's Society.

Ballard, C. (2005) 'Drugs used to relieve behavioural symptoms in people with dementia or an unacceptable chemical cosh?' *International Psychogeriatrics*, 17 (1): 4–12.

Bullock, R. (2002) *Building a Modern Service*, St Albans: Altman Publishing.

Cohen-Mansfield, J. (2000) 'Approaches to the Management of Disruptive Behaviors', in R. Rubinstein and M.P. Lawton (eds), *Alzheimer's Disease and Related Dementias: Strategies Care and Research*, New York: Springer Publishing Company.

Cummings, J., Mega, M., Gray, K., Rosenberg-Thompson, S., Carusi, D. and Gornbein, J. (1994) 'The neuropsychiatric inventory: a comprehensive assessment of psychopathology in dementia', *Neurology*, 44: 2308–14.

Dempsey, O.P. and Moore, H. (2005) 'Psychotropic prescribing for older people in residential care in the UK, are guidelines being followed?' *Primary Care and Community Psychiatry*, 10 (1): 13–18.

Department of Health (2009) *Living well with dementia: National Dementia Strategy*, London: Department of Health.

Folstein, M.F., Folstein, S. and McHugh, P. (1975) 'Mini-mental State. A practical guide for grading the cognitive state of patients for the clinician', *Journal of Psychiatric Research*, 12: 189–98.

Fossey, J. and James, I. (2008) *Evidence-based approaches for improving dementia care in care homes*, London: Alzheimer's Society.

Gill, S.S., Rochon, P.A., Herrmann, N., Lee, P.E., Sykora, K., Gunraj, N., Normand, S.T., Gurwitz, J.H., Marras, C., Wodchis, W.P. and Mamdani, M. (2005) 'Atypical antipsychotic drugs and risk of ischaemic stroke: population based retrospective cohort study', *British Medical Journal*, 330 (7489): 445.

Howard, R., Ballard, C., O'Brien, J. and Burns, A. (2001) 'Guidelines for the management of agitation in dementia', *International Journal Geriatric Psychiatry*, 16: 714–17.

James, I.A., Reichelt, F.K., Freeston, M. and Barton, S. (2007) 'Schema as memories: Implications for treatment', *Journal of Cognitive Psychotherapy: An international quarterly*, 21 (1): 51–57.

James, I.A. and Stephenson, M. (2007) 'Behaviour that challenges us: the Newcastle support model', *Journal of Dementia Care*, 15 (5): 19–22.

James, I.A., Stephenson, M., Mackenzie, L. and Roe, P. (2006) 'Dealing with challenging behaviour through an analysis of need: the Colombo approach', in M. Marshall (ed.), *On the Move: Walking not Wandering*, London: Hawker Press.

James, I.A., Wood-Mitchell, A. and Waterworth, A. (2006) 'Treating Challenging Behaviour in Dementia with Psychotropic Medication – help or hindrance?', *Psychology Special Interest Group for Older People (PSIGE) Newsletter*, BPS: 93.

Keady, J., Clarke, C.L., Wilkinson, H., Gibb, G.E., Williams, L., Luce, A. and Cook, A. (2009) 'Alcohol-related brain damage: Narrative storylines and risk constructions', *Health, Risk and Society*, 11 (4): 321–40.

Kitwood. T. (1997) *Dementia reconsidered: the person comes first*, Buckingham: Open University Press.

Macdonald, A.J.D., Carpenter, G.I., Box, O., Roberts, A. and Sahu, S. (2002) 'Dementia and use of psychotropic medication in non-Elderly Mentally Infirm nursing home in South East England', *Age and Ageing*, 31: 58–64.

McGrath, A.M. and Jackson, G.A. (1996) 'Survey of neuroleptic prescribing in residents of nursing homes in Glasgow', *British Medical Journal*, 312 (7031): 611–12.

Mackenzie, L., Wood-Mitchell, A. and James, I.A. (2007) 'Guidelines on the use of dolls in care settings', *Journal of Dementia Care*, 15 (1): 26–27.

McShane, R., Keene, J., Gedling, K., Fairburn, C., Jacoby, R. and Hope, T. (1997) 'Do neuroleptic drugs hasten cognitive decline in dementia?' *British Medical Journal*, 314 (7076): 266–70.

Moniz-Cook, E.R., Woods, R. and Gardiner, E. (2000) 'Staff factors associated with perception of behaviour as 'challenging' in residential and nursing homes', *Aging & Mental Health*, 4 (1): 48–55.

National Institute for Health and Clinical Excellence/Social Care Institute for Excellence (2006) *Dementia: supporting people with dementia and their carers in health and social care. NICE clinical practice guideline 42*, London: National Institute for Health and Clinical Excellence.

Sink, K.M., Holden, F.H. and Yaffe, K. (2004) 'Pharmacological treatment of neuropsychiatric symptoms of dementia: A review of the evidence', *Journal of the American Medical Association*, 293 (5): 596–608.

Smith, K., Milburn, M. and Mackenzie, L. (2008) '"Poor command of English": Is it a problem in care homes? If so, what can be done about it?' *Journal of Dementia Care*, 16 (6): 37–38.

Wood-Mitchell, A., James, I.A., Waterworth, A. and Swann, A. (2008) 'Factors influencing the prescribing of medications by old age psychiatrists for behavioural and psychological symptoms of dementia: a qualitative study', *Age and Ageing*, 3: 1–16.

Wood-Mitchell, A., Mackenzie, L., Stephenson, M. and James, I.A. (2007) 'Treating challenging behaviour in care settings: audit of a community service using the neuropsychiatric inventory', *PSIGE Newsletter*, British Psychological Society, 101: 19–23.

10 Later life liaison services

Delivering holistic care in a general hospital setting

Helen Pratt and Lorraine Burgess

Key messages

- A complex overlap of mental health and physical health problems is very common in older people who are in-patients in general hospitals.
- Collaborative working relationships with the general hospital, at all levels of the organisation, are essential for the delivery of liaison services.
- Liaison Practitioners' whole focus is on the promotion of person-centred care, through direct consultation with patients and their families or by indirect consultation influencing the care delivered by the general hospital staff.
- Education and training are essential components of Liaison Services' model of care.

Introduction

The aim of this chapter is to demonstrate the application of an holistic mental health model of care within interdisciplinary general hospital settings. It will highlight literature summarising the prevalence of mental health needs in general hospitals, examine Later Life Liaison Services and discuss key policy drivers.

A composite case study, based on examples of care taken from a number of anonymised patient cases will be utilised. This will enable the authors to discuss their own assessment approaches and interventions. The composite case study highlights the importance of a person-centred approach and provides discussion of emerging themes. The chapter will also consider the difficulties encountered by non-mental health care staff in caring for the older person with mental health needs. Examples of care successes and dilemmas are used by the authors to reflect the most prevalent model of service provision for Later Life Liaison Services: that of single liaison practitioners working holistically within interdisciplinary general hospital settings.

Liaison Services involve the provision of dedicated specialist mental health staff time within the general hospital. Liaison staff undertake comprehensive mental health assessments (with the older person and their carers), care planning, treatment reviews, discharge planning and signposting or referring patients to mental health services. In addition, these services provide advice and guide the general hospital staff in their care delivery through the provision of education and training.

The challenge for liaison services

The number of older people with different types of mental health problems is predicted to increase. It is estimated that the number of people with dementia will have doubled in 30 years (Alzheimer's Society 2007, McCrone *et al.* 2008).

Older people occupy two-thirds of general hospital beds, with a large number presenting with mental health problems. This population also tend to have longer stays in the general hospital, with intense care episodes and multiple contacts with different staff, and are most likely to experience significant morbidity and mortality (Holmes and House 2000, Royal College of Psychiatrists 2005, Academy of Medical Royal Colleges 2008). In recent years, there have been a number of damning reports of the care of older people in general hospitals. These reports commented on poor care delivery with regard to dignity and malnutrition (Health Advisory Service 1998, Age Concern 2006, Fielding and Craig 2007). The Audit Commission and Healthcare Commission (2006) highlighted older people's concerns about the loss of dignity for people with dementia as a result of care and treatment received when admitted to hospital for a physical illness. Examples included meals being taken away before being eaten, the use of restraints and care practices which increase disorientation, such as spending time in inappropriate clothing and experiencing repeated ward moves. In the United Kingdom (UK) policy guidance states:

> Due to the very common nature of mental illness in later life, and its co-morbidity with physical conditions, the majority of mild and moderate severity mental illness will be managed in mainstream settings, by staff without psychiatric training.
>
> (Department of Health 2005: 3)

However, evidence suggests that general hospital staff lack the confidence, knowledge base and skills to assess, treat and care for older people with mental health needs (Academy of Medical Royal Colleges 2008). Mayou (2007) found that despite increasing awareness of the emotional and behavioural aspects of physical illness, Liaison Services have yet to achieve substantial influence and have had only modest effects on the delivery of medical care by physicians and other specialists. Holmes, Bentley and Cameron (2002), in a survey of 210 mental health services for older people across all general hospitals in the UK concluded that in a majority of cases liaison services had been provided by either medical staff or single liaison practitioners.

Despite the reality of co-existing mental and physical health care needs, an organisational split between acute care and mental health services has developed (Academy of Medical Royal Colleges 2008). A consensus statement issued by the Mental Health and Older People Forum (2008) attributes the development of separate commissioning and management structures to the lack of any additional targeted investment or clear performance indicators for liaison services. Mental health trusts have focused their work on the community population. Thus patients with mental health needs in a general hospital are not prioritised (Royal College of Psychiatrists 2005, National Audit Office 2007, Academy of Medical Royal Colleges 2008). Increasingly, there is a view amongst general hospital staff that mental health problems in older people are a problem for mental health services, despite the fact that these patients are under their care and that, whilst in-patients, they do not have access to these same mental health services. Mental health problems are therefore either not detected, or if they are detected are often treated sub-optimally (Royal College of Psychiatrists 2005).

The Care Quality Commission (2008) assesses the progress of health service providers in meeting core and developmental *Standards for Better Health*. In the future, this may well be a means by which general hospitals are held to account if they have failed to implement the national guidance as set out in the *National Service Framework for Mental Health* (Department of Health 1999) and the National Institute for Health and Clinical Excellence (2005), as required within Core Standard C5 (Care Quality Commission 2008).

These are the challenges that have become 'a call to arms' for the development of Later Life Liaison Services in general hospitals. The emphasis now, when developing these services, is on ensuring that the general hospital staff is supported to develop the skills to assess, treat and manage the more routine cases, and knows how to refer to mental health services when more complex presentations arise.

Policy considerations

Various UK Government and college reports (Department of Health 2001, Royal College of Physicians and Royal College of Psychiatrists 2003, National Audit Office 2007, Department of Health 2008) stress the importance of access to psychological care for people with physical conditions and mental health needs. In addition, the National Audit Office (2007) identified dementia care as core work for geriatricians within general hospitals and that theirs is a key role in its assessment and management, as well as identifying the presence of acute confusional state (delirium). The ICD-10 diagnostic classification of delirium (acute confusion) (World Health Organization 1993) is:

- Impairment of consciousness and attention.
- Global disturbance of cognition (perceptual distortions, impairment of abstract thinking, recall and recent memory, and distortion of time).
- Psychomotor disturbance (hypo- or hyperactivity).
- Disturbance of sleep-wake cycle.
- Emotional disturbances (depression, anxiety, irritability or euphoria).
- Rapid onset and fluctuations of symptoms over the course of the day.

It has long been recognised that the attitudes, skills and knowledge of staff working with people with dementia (and other mental health problems) have the potential to influence the person's well-being, quality of life and function (National Institute for Health and Clinical Excellence/Social Care Institute for Excellence 2006). NICE/SCIE also noted that organisational constraints and obstacles must be addressed in order for education and training to bring about the necessary change. Fielding and Craig (2007) and the Academy of Medical Royal Colleges (2008) take this argument further by requiring general hospitals to have a mechanism for executive boards to receive regular updates on their whole organisation strategy to address skills and training deficits in relation to the care of older people with mental health needs.

Key government reports and NICE guidance have attempted to provide direction for commissioners and service providers with regard to the unmet needs of older people experiencing mental health problems in general hospitals (Department of Health 2001, 2005, 2009, National Audit Office 2007). Recommendations include: proposals for discharge processes for patients with dementia (Health and Social Care Change Agent Team 2003); standards for education and training for general hospital staff; guidance on the development and implementation of protocols or pathways for the care of older people with dementia, delirium and depression, as well as the management of self-harm, violence and aggression for all ages presenting at the general hospital (National Institute for Health and Clinical Excellence 2004, 2005, 2007a, 2007b, National Institute for Health and Clinical Excellence/Social Care Institute for Excellence 2006).

Models of care

The liaison service model of care differs from the typical model of mental health service care delivery, in that general hospital staff deliver the majority of care. Thus, mental health staff within liaison services work on influencing the care delivery by general hospital staff through the act and process of liaison (Roberts 2002, Sharrock *et al.* 2006). The fundamental principle is the importance of establishing and maintaining collaborative working relationships between professionals, services and organisations: liaison is a strategy or process and not an end in itself. The provision of person-centred direct patient consultation continues to remain a component of the liaison model of care, that is mental health assessment and delivery of psychotherapeutic interventions by trained liaison practitioners themselves. However, the emphasis now within later life liaison services is on the development and maintenance of working relationships with interdisciplinary general hospital staff, as this has had the greatest impact on the delivery of holistic care.

Person-centred care needs to be the bedrock underpinning any collaborative liaison model of care (Minshull 2007). Liaison practitioners work to establish and maintain relationships with the general hospital staff based on respect, promotion of self-worth and a focus on the team's strengths and abilities. Indirectly this enables the promotion of person-hood of the patients for whom they are caring. The liaison model of care also needs to include direct and indirect clinical and organisational consultation (Roberts 2002). Regardless of the numbers of practitioners, or range of professional disciplines working within a liaison service, the model of care needs to address four key areas:

1   Direct consultation – the patient is directly involved with every stage of assessment and management.
2   Indirect consultation – this targets the delivery of care by the hospital team: practical care delivery, role modelling, effective communication with patients, informal education and the provision of written resources.
3   Organisational consultation – the development of protocols, guidelines and policies at a ward, department or whole hospital level, covering quality of care, access to services, and service evaluation.
4   Collaborative working – the formation of alliances, establishing links between knowledge and practice, and enabling the provision of formal education.

Despite having different commissioning and service provision arrangements, the focus of work for the authors has been the development of collaborative working relationships within and across the general hospital. One of the authors was employed by mental health services to work as a liaison nurse in the general hospital, alongside the equivalent of two sessions from a consultant psychiatrist. The other author was both employed by and worked within the general hospital as a dementia specialist nurse, again with very limited provision of consultant psychiatric time from the local NHS Mental Health Trust.

It is interesting to note that a majority of Liaison Services (for all ages) are commissioned by NHS Mental Health Trusts. Indeed, in their review of liaison services, Roberts and Whitehead (2002) found that 44 percent were employed by NHS Mental Health Trusts and 22 percent were employed by the acute sector, in their review of liaison services.

Applying principles

This section utilises a composite case study to depict the process of referral, assessment, intervention and management by the liaison practitioners with general hospital staff. It reflects direct and indirect liaison, as the later life Liaison Service model of care delivery.

Referral

Case Study A. The liaison practitioner receives a written referral asking for capacity assessment and discharge advice for Elsie, an 83-year-old lady on a medical ward. The referral states that she has a previously-diagnosed vascular dementia, lives alone in sheltered accommodation and was found 10 days ago, prior to admission, by the warden, collapsed at home. Elsie has declined treatment for a urine infection on the ward. There has been some aggression towards staff providing care and she is refusing to go into 24-hour care.

Care delivery in relation to case study A

After a telephone conversation with the ward, the Liaison Practitioner agrees to an assessment of Elsie, as there are risks pertaining to her refusal of treatment. Over the telephone, the Liaison Practitioner directs the ward nurses to contact Elsie's general practitioner (GP), mental health services, warden and family, in order to establish what is known about her. The Liaison Practitioner guides staff with the sorts of questions to ask in relation to any changes in her mental health, functioning and risk issues when she is at home. A nurse is to obtain information with regard to Elsie's life history and values: for example, what are her views on taking medication?

The ward nurses obtain the following information regarding Elsie: she has a very close friend called Bob, who was her neighbour, but he moved into 24-hour care five months ago. Bob's son, who visits Elsie regularly both on the ward and at her home, reports that, other than himself, Elsie has no other next of kin, friends or formal support. Bob and Elsie had previously played an active role in the Salvation Army for most of their lives. Bob's son states that Elsie had been managing very well until Bob went into care. Since then she has become tearful, more forgetful and her appetite has decreased. She has never been aggressive, was compliant with her medication, and was not normally as confused as she appears on the ward. Elsie is not open to mental health services.

Emerging themes

A referral to Liaison Services frequently does not reflect the underlying patient complexities (Longson 2007). All too often the referral is driven by the general hospital's focus on capacity or discharge (placement into care in this example), and does not relate to the patient's or family's views. A number of Liaison Services have developed referral forms in order to deal with this ongoing problem.

However, Roberts and Whitehead (2002) found that formal referral processes deterred hospital teams from referring and seeking help. As evidence to date reflects a pattern of under-referral into mental health services by general hospitals (Royal College of Psychiatrists 2005), this potential barrier needs to be considered when establishing Liaison Services. The authors found that effective liaison was encouraged by offering daily designated times for telephone discussion which were open to any professional general hospital staff member or patient's relative, in addition to a formal referral process.

Asking the general hospital staff to obtain the patient's life history as well as other mental health and risk information was intended to develop their understanding of the value of person-centred assessment. This will enable the staff to begin to understand that some of Elsie's refusal of care may be as a result of her deteriorating physical health, losses, difficulties with memory and orientation while in a strange environment – the hospital ward. It would help avoid hasty decisions about capacity and discharge. They would also get to know more about her life and thereby start to engage with her as a person.

Proactive collaborative liaison about the referral process with the whole hospital system is fundamental to Later Life Liaison Services. The authors' experience is that for the first six months at least this needs to run in parallel with the provision of ward-based assessments by the liaison practitioner. A focus on organisational consultation is required. For example, each ward or service needs to understand, with case illustrations, how a Liaison referral would benefit their patients and the staff team. This should include briefings with the wider management team, such as duty senior operational managers, pre-operative departments and allied health professionals.

Assessment, discussion and intervention

Case Study B. When the Liaison Practitioner arrives on the ward to assess Elsie, the nurses state that she will not take any medication and is aggressive, which they consider to be due to her dementia. They have asked the OT to complete a Mini-mental State Examination (Folstein, Folstein and McHugh 1975) and she scored 6/30. They think that a medical ward is not the right place for her and she needs to go into an EMI home.

Care delivery in relation to case study B

The Liaison Practitioner spends some time observing Elsie while she interacts with ward staff, then reviews the medical notes, blood results, medication compliance and nursing care records. The Practitioner completes a mental health and risk assessment with Elsie, in a quiet room on the ward. The Liaison Practitioner advises the junior doctor and nurses that the assessment suggests that Elsie appears to be presenting with a delirium with paranoid ideation, in addition to her vascular dementia. She may also be experiencing depression, although it is too early to assess the extent of the depression whilst delirium is clouding the picture.

The Liaison Practitioner explains the diagnosis to Elsie, with a nurse present, so that the nursing team know what has been said, and can remind Elsie of this. The Liaison Practitioner provides the multi-disciplinary care team (MDT) with evidence-based written information about the care of patients with delirium, dementia and associated symptoms. The Liaison Practitioner also talks through the importance of Elsie remaining in hospital, staying on the current ward, so that she can be supported to accept treatment for the infection.

The Liaison Practitioner is invited to attend the ward MDT meeting, with the Consultant Physician present. The Liaison Practitioner encourages discussion within the meeting as to when 'a refusal is a refusal', in relation to Elsie's refusal of medication for her infection. Discussion focuses on the importance of not assuming that this refusal means Elsie is declining to accept treatment or help, as she may not understand what she is declining or the consequences. The Liaison Practitioner highlights all practical steps to be undertaken in order to help Elsie make an informed decision, in accordance with the five principles of the *Mental Capacity Act* (2005):

1 Every adult has the right to make his or her own decisions and must be assumed to have capacity to make them unless it is proved otherwise.
2 A person must be given all practicable help before anyone treats them as not being able to make their own decisions.
3 Just because an individual makes what might be seen as an unwise decision, they should not be treated as lacking capacity to make that decision.
4 Anything done or any decision made on behalf of a person who lacks capacity must be done in their best interests.
5 Anything done for or on behalf of a person who lacks capacity should be the least restrictive of their basic rights and freedoms.

The Liaison Practitioner also asked the MDT to review Elsie's medication and its administration:

- What is essential? What could be discontinued in the short term, while she is suspicious of taking medication on the ward?
- Can administration be reduced to twice daily?
- Is a syrup form of medication available?
- Is medication more acceptable to Elsie if administered by different staff?
- Can administration be timed flexibly for when she is more settled and lucid?

A staged management plan is clearly documented by the Liaison Practitioner in the medical and nursing notes, with a review date and guidance on when to contact the Practitioner. The Liaison Practitioner agrees to provide brief frequent reviews of Elsie on the medical ward.

Emerging themes

Gill, Rigatelli and Ferrari (2007) and Steis and Fick (2008) reported on the poor detection of delirium by the general hospital medical and nursing staff. The Royal College of Psychiatrists (2005) identified that general hospitals do not systematically consider the possibility of delirium at admission, or of its development whilst the person is in hospital, despite extensive literature advocating the identification of predisposing factors for the development of delirium (Inouye *et. al.* 1993, Inouye 2000). Steis and Fick (2008) found that to improve recognition by nurses, they must have time to spend with the patient in order to learn how to recognise delirium's fluctuating course. They also identified the importance of inter-shift handover, to ensure seamless care. Differing professional perspectives are also important, so MDT discussion of the patient's clinical presentation has a valuable role.

Episodes of delirium occur so frequently in a general hospital that a liaison service cannot be directly involved with all cases. Therefore, there is a major role for education, training and collaborative working (Gill, Rigatelli and Ferrari 2007). The Liaison Practitioner has a role in trying to focus the general hospital's delivery of care beyond preoccupations with risk avoidance and narrow interpretations of situations and information.

The culture of cognitive testing and assessment has a major impact on the person with dementia (Cheston and Bender 2000), through the expectations of other staff in response to evidence of cognitive impairment. It is vital that Liaison Practitioners highlight these issues. The Liaison Practitioner has a role in helping to develop the concept that recovery is more than the traditional biomedical notion, and rather is an 'attempt to understand people's experiences in the broader context of their lives' (Berzins 2004: 4).

Principles of recovery can be applied to people with mental health problems, including those experiencing cognitive impairment (Keady and Hardman 2010). Moreover, there is too much naïve interpretation of the results of cognitive tests. All too often the scores from brief, poorly administered screening assessments are utilised to make decisions about future long-term placement and discharge. Liaison Practitioners need to ensure there is cautious interpretation of these formal tests within the general hospital and that a person-centred approach is what underpins the holistic assessment and intervention process.

Challenging behaviour

Case Study C. On one of the review visits by the Liaison Practitioner, the nurses report that Elsie is at the nurses' station or door, and when they try to get her to sit at her bedside she is verbally aggressive with them.

Care delivery in relation to case study C

The Liaison Practitioner suggests that the nurse observes a review assessment, subject to Elsie's agreement, in order to establish how Elsie perceives her problems. There are a number of reasons for this:

- To model communication skills.
- For the staff team to hear Elsie's own words and views.
- For staff to realise that time spent now will enable a trusting therapeutic relationship with Elsie to be built.

The intention is to enable them to see the person behind the diagnosis of delirium and dementia, thereby positively impacting on their care delivery. During the interview Elsie reveals that she feels scared by the other patients, as one lady shouts at her; Elsie wants to help the nurses as she believes she works on the ward; and Elsie is tearful when talking about her flat and Bob. Following the interview, the observing nurse states her surprise at how articulate Elsie was and that staff had not realised how frightened she had been.

Emerging themes

Developing the skills to communicate with people with mental health needs is often an onerous responsibility, as they far exceed those required in the normal routines of daily life. Some nurses, particularly those who lack knowledge in dementia care, may feel this responsibility is too great (Packer 1999). Packer (1999) suggests that caring for a person with dementia takes a particular type of person, with few staff having the tolerance, compassion and empathy required to fulfil this role. It could be argued that, particularly given the numbers of frail elderly in general hospital settings, all nurses should possess these skills regardless of area of work. The feelings of helplessness a person with dementia often exhibits can be transferred to staff, who may then feel unable to empathise or relieve the patient's distress.

This is especially evident when the patient is exhibiting behaviour perceived by staff as challenging. Woods (2001) has recommended that behaviour should be seen as a form of communication, which is being used to express unmet needs. This need to communicate through behaviour is frequently unrecognised by general hospital staff, where instead the patient is perceived as a 'problem'. Education and training in relation to understanding behaviour may aid in rectifying this situation and play a vital role in liaison.

The development of a relationship is the primary vehicle of care in psychiatry (Peplau 1964). In the setting of liaison, this relationship is with the patient (and family, as appropriate), but also with the care team on the general hospital ward. Forming therapeutic alliances will have the most successful outcomes for the patient.

The Liaison Practitioner has a role in conveying the importance of attachment, its implications for the maintenance of existing relationships whilst the person is admitted to hospital, with proactive communication, and the establishment of new attachments with the ward team.

Problems with nutrition

Case Study D. On one of the review visits by the Liaison Practitioner, the nurses state that Elsie is declining to eat some of the meals at her bedside and is refusing to allow them to assist her to eat and drink. Some of the staff report that they have 'had enough of problem behaviour with Elsie and she needs to move to a mental health ward'.

Care delivery in relation to case study D

The Liaison Practitioner discusses with the nursing team factors that may be causing Elsie not to eat and drink. Elsie is 'on the go' walking around the ward all the time.

The Liaison Practitioner explores a number of possibilities for the change in her dietary intake: Elsie may believe she is on the ward to help, reflecting her belief that she is there as a nursing assistant, as this was her job years ago; paranoia or distress symptoms may remain from her dementia and subsiding delirium; loss of appetite may be associated with depression; or she may feel a lack of dignity in eating at her bedside.

Other issues such as the effect of medication and poor physical health are considered. The Liaison Practitioner identifies various alternative care delivery techniques for trial to see if these help and a staged plan for the MDT to follow is documented in the notes:

- Encourage Elsie to join the nursing assistants when they sit down for a break as this may fit in with her belief she is 'at work'.

- Offer finger food that Elsie can 'eat on the go'.
- Offer small amounts more frequently, as opposed to a large plate at set meal times.
- Ask Bob's son to purchase things Elsie likes as he used to do this for her when she was at home.
- Ensure good quality food presentation.
- Introduce a social atmosphere more conducive to eating – which may mean sitting at a dining table, away from her bed, with other patients.
- Include the ward clerk and other team members to help with observations of Elsie if she is up and walking around the ward, particularly at busy times for the nursing staff. More staff may not be needed to undertake observations at a distance, if a plan is agreed by the whole ward team.

The nurses are to monitor her intake over a number of days with diet and fluid charts, weigh Elsie and review her Malnutrition Universal Screening Tool score (BAPEN 2003).

The general hospital has recruited volunteers as an additional ward resource to assist with meal times and has introduced a 'red tray' initiative to ensure that vulnerable patients with nutritional needs are identified and supported. Over the following weeks, Elsie continues to recover from the infection and delirium. The care strategies that the nurses have adopted result in Elsie becoming more settled, she has begun to eat and drink at an acceptable level, and interacts more with the staff.

Emerging themes

The quote below reflects a common lack of understanding of behaviour that is seen in general hospitals:

> ... hospital staff sometimes interpreted behaviour such as wandering off, as evidence that the person was refusing or avoiding [care] ... hospitals were inflexible in not understanding or allowing for the problems of fear and confusion that can be problematic for people with dementia.
>
> (Nuffield Council on Bioethics 2009: 52)

The Liaison Practitioner can have the greatest impact here with the use of indirect consultation. This involves informal MDT discussions, brief ward-based educational sessions and provision of written nursing care guidance, all aimed at focusing the ward team on the importance of seeing behaviour as a form of communication. This enables the ward team to begin to understand why behaviour is occurring and develop action care strategies to minimise it themselves. Age Concern (2006) found that six out of 10 older people become malnourished in a general hospital, with people over 80 years five times more likely to develop malnutrition: 'people with dementia were not receiving adequate or sensitive help with eating, as a result of which, meals were being taken away uneaten' (Healthcare Commission 2007: 29).

The Care Quality Commission (2008) reviews general hospitals against the core standards for better health in relation to dignity and nutrition. Key recommendations were the importance of wards having protected meal times, offering a choice of meals, and providing patients with assistance with food and drink (Healthcare Commission 2007). The Healthcare Commission review also found that not all NHS Trusts were monitoring the issue of nutritional needs of patients and whether these were being met by current care practices. As nutritional issues are so important for patients with mental health needs in a general hospital, Liaison Practitioners need to work collaboratively with Trust leads or nutritional steering groups. A very positive example for one of the Liaison Practitioners has been involvement in the training of general hospital volunteers as they start with the trust, to increase their understanding of mental health issues. These volunteers are recruited as an additional resource to assist with meal times.

Within dementia care there has been an emerging evidence base supporting non-pharmacological assessment and management of behaviour and psychological problems (Kitwood 1997, Stokes 2000, National Institute for Health and Clinical Excellence/Social Care Institute for Excellence 2006, Fossey and James 2008). Liaison Practitioners are utilising this emerging evidence and applying it to the general hospital setting. The focus of the training sessions that both Liaison Practitioners have been delivering to all professional disciplines within the general hospital has been the development of a psychological model of the understanding of behaviour.

Discharge planning

Case Study E. The nurses express concern about how safe Elsie would be if she were to return home, as she has been saying that she wants to go back to the flat to be with Bob. She has said that she does not need any help when back home.

Care delivery in relation to case study E

The Liaison Practitioner discusses with Elsie where she wants to live and where 'home' is, over a number of the reviews on the ward. This changes from Elsie being adamant about returning to her flat, to living with Bob, and on other occasions to 'being with the Salvation Army'. Over a two-week period Elsie says that she 'wishes to be cared for, like they are doing for her in hospital'. Given that the Salvation Army had been such a large part of her life, the option of living in one of their residential homes is put to Elsie, at the suggestion of the hospital chaplain in discussion with the Liaison Practitioner. The hospital social worker provides written information and asks the manager of one of the homes to come and speak to Elsie about it. Arrangements are put in place and she is accepted by the home.

The ward nurses report that Elsie has become a 'delayed discharge' as she is medically fit for discharge, but no bed is available in the care home. They request that Elsie be transferred to an interim care home to avoid delaying discharge. Elsie had declined this when asked by the nurses. The Liaison Practitioner acts as an advocate on behalf of Elsie that this would not be in her best interests, stating it would cause her further distress and potentially result in deterioration in her mental health. There is agreement that she remain in hospital, on the same ward, until her discharge to the Salvation Army home. The Liaison Practitioner provides a written summary for the GP and care home, with a brief version of this for Elsie.

Emerging themes

The Royal College of Psychiatrists (2005) suggests that Liaison Practitioners are best placed to facilitate discharge planning when there are a number of risks and uncertainty around risks at home. General hospital staff may make decisions that reflect defensive practice when it comes to discharging older people with confusion. Placement in care is often the solution to this, without any consideration that there may be as many, if not more, risks associated with going into care, for the person him/herself. Our experience is that the liaison practitioner's role is often to lead decision-making that involves risks in relation to an older person with mental health needs.

Risk assessment and risk management planning need to be proportionate to the perceived risks and involve the person with mental health needs and their family (Royal College of Psychiatrists 2008). The Academy of Medical Royal Colleges (2008) highlights the need for general hospital staff to have training in assessing and managing risk. The Health and Social Care Change Agent Team (2003) provided guidance for general hospitals in facilitating seamless discharges for older people with dementia. This required all trusts to have a named person, with dementia expertise, responsible for discharge co-ordination and that all discharge decisions be made by an interdisciplinary team led by a person trained in addressing the needs of people with dementia.

Whilst Liaison Practitioners are sometimes called upon to assist with discharge planning, invariably the authors have found that this is when the issue of the patient's capacity to agree to a care placement has arisen. There were good examples of the ward team proactively liaising with community mental health teams; however, there have also been a large number of occasions where discharge decisions and planning did not involve mental health services, families or even the person him/herself.

The issue of 'delayed discharge' has become a contentious one, following the *Community Care (Delayed Discharges) Act* (Department of Health 2003). In a study of delayed discharges by Hughes *et al.* (2007), it was found that patients with cognitive impairment were almost twice as likely to experience a delay in their discharge as well as being more likely to be discharged to a care home. A report by the Alzheimer's Society (2007) suggested that delayed discharges for people with dementia are problematic, not just for the person and family, but also for policy-makers, as they lead to inefficient and inequitable use of resources, i.e. acute hospital beds. Resolving these tensions is complex. Hughes *et al.* (2007) recommended the provision of interim beds outside the general hospital, in order to avoid delays in the patient remaining in a general hospital bed until they are placed in a care home permanently. Whilst a move to a temporary placement relieves the problem for the general hospital in its use of resources, it can result in increased dependency for patients temporarily placed in care homes. This can impact on rehabilitation options, particularly for people with dementia. Moreover, the National Audit Office (2007) report has highlighted evidence that people with dementia were most often in acute hospital beds and most no longer needed to be there, but intermediate care services were reluctant to admit people with dementia and there was a lack of resources and alternatives. Decisions such as moving into a care home are associated with any number of psychological and emotional factors for the person him/herself and often need to be taken over time. All too often 'time' is the precious resource that general hospitals do not have to offer the older person.

In conclusion, the focus of this Applying Principles section has been that person-centred care needs to be the bedrock underpinning any liaison model of care. The composite case study and exploration of the emerging themes demonstrate the importance of the overlapping role of the core principles of the liaison model of care: direct and indirect clinical and organisational consultation, bound together by the process of liaison (Roberts 2002). These underpin any Later Life Liaison Service, whether this be a lone

Practitioner, or a whole Mental Health Liaison Team. Effective Liaison Services build alliances, support teams, challenge practice and enable the integration of knowledge into practice; these all result in improved quality of care for the patient.

Discussion

The authors have used examples of care successes and dilemmas, to reflect the person-centred model in Later Life Liaison Services. A number of emerging themes, briefly debated within the case study examples, highlight the central role that indirect consultation played in the model of service provision, as well as the value of creative problem solving with the ward teams in order to address the care needs (in our example) of a person with dementia. The focus of indirect consultation was to positively influence the quality of the care delivery by the general hospital staff.

Sharrock *et al.* (2006) undertook a survey of general hospital nurses, who said that they were not prepared for mental health needs. That is, they lacked the knowledge, skills or confidence, and lacked expert assistance and work place policies, to support them in delivering care. This problem is increased when patient behaviour is perceived as difficult, threatening or disruptive. Fundamentally, the focus of the work of the Liaison Practitioner, as illustrated by the case study, is in directing the care delivery of others. There has been limited guidance or evidence as to how Liaison Practitioners can best develop the necessary skills. As the case study around nutritional issues shows, the work involves having the skills to work both with individual staff and with organisational systems (see also Ragaisis 2005). Liaison Practitioners essentially require the attitude, philosophical principles, personal attributes and approach to focus on relationship building at all levels in an organisation. For the authors, this involved 'getting to know' the staff teams, taking the time to build and maintain relationships with ward clerks, volunteers, professional staff, business and training managers. At a system level, this mirrors the individual work of 'getting to know' the person behind the mental health presentation, which Liaison Practitioners seek to support the general hospital staff in undertaking themselves, with their patients. The case study highlights the time commitment the Liaison Practitioner must make in reviewing the patient and in maintaining the confidence and competencies of the ward staff in care delivery.

Debates over the place of single practitioners in delivering Liaison Services have been rolling on for some time. The Academy of Medical Royal Colleges (2008) and the Royal College of Psychiatrists (2005) highlight the tendency for rapid burnout, and that services can be prone to collapse without notice. McNamara *et al.*'s (2008) survey of consultation-liaison nurses in Australia found that lack of supervision, support and resources, lack of political influence and increased workload capacity all negatively affected sole practitioners' satisfaction with the role. There are certainly times when lack of support and isolation impact heavily on the sole practitioner.

One way to address this is to look for support from other sole practitioners in Liaison Services; this peer support is something that the authors have been undertaking for some years, with each other. Having the time agreed from local managers to attend and be involved in the National Liaison events was also a valuable support. The authors also found that undertaking some joint educational initiatives, for example a joint conference for World Mental Health and World Alzheimer's Day was a great way to pool resources, expertise and time, whilst providing a well-received educational day for around 200 general hospital staff.

The Department of Health (2009) recognises that clinicians themselves are best placed to work as partners and leaders in order to focus on improving individual skills, organisational systems and the whole quality of NHS care. The authors established an informal regional network in order to support the large number of sole Liaison Practitioners locally. This network delivered a regional conference to stakeholders and commissioners focusing on the importance of establishing Liaison Services, developed a business case that was presented to the educational leads from the Strategic Health Authority, developed guidance in the form of a checklist for the establishment of Liaison Services that was adopted by CSIP North West (Pratt and Ratcliffe 2005), and collaborated with the sharing of operational policies and pathways or protocols.

The authors found that there were both advantages and disadvantages to their employment and management arrangements sitting within either the acute trust or mental health trust, as highlighted in Table 10.1.

Both practitioners found that there were ways to try to overcome some of these disadvantages; however, these took up a large amount of organisational consultation time, and thus impacted on time available for direct and indirect work. This demonstrated the importance of peer support for sole Liaison Practitioners, as the journey to develop improved quality of care can seem a very lonely one. The Liaison Practitioner's role also extends to promoting the role of governance structures in responding to concerns over poor care delivery, and in tying new developments into care pathways and Trust educational and training priorities.

Reference has been made throughout this chapter to the central role that education and training play, which also reflects key policy directives (Department of Health 2001, Royal College of Psychiatrists 2005, National Institute for Health and Clinical Excellence/ Social Care Institute for Excellence 2006, Age Concern 2006, Healthcare Commission

Table 10.1 Advantages and disadvantages of employment and management arrangements

Employed by and responsible to an acute trust		Employed by and responsible to a mental health trust	
Advantages	*Disadvantages*	*Advantages*	*Disadvantages*
Get to know the staff – provides a sense of belonging	Trust not realising the huge scope of the role	Line management from mental health services	Unable to access resources, e.g. to assist with training
Feeling valued and committed to develop services	Lack of clinical supervision within trust	Access to clinical supervision from mental health trust	Governance issues fall between both trusts in relation to patient incidences
Knowing the structure of the organisation, e.g. being able to access training resources	Limited cross-trusts (mental health and acute) joint working	Peer support from other liaison practitioners, e.g. working age, alcohol	Limited cross-trusts (mental health and acute) joint working
Being seen as an expert for the trust	Trust wanting unrealistic immediate results	Support from senior managers in driving forward liaison service development	Lack of ownership of the issues by acute trust
Focusing on how targets can be realistically achieved from within the trust	No direct access to refer into mental health services	Direct access referral into mental health services and access to patient data	Limited understanding of structures and organisation of acute trust

2007, Academy of Medical Royal Colleges 2008, Department of Health 2008, 2009). Evidence has started to emerge on what educational strategies need to address for Liaison (Royal College of Psychiatrists 2005, Lloyd and Guthrie 2007). However, Minshull (2007) identified that the skill set needed to provide care for older people is significantly different from skills required to care for adults of working age. The approach needs to be creative and flexible, with the identification of core competencies for all general hospital staff in caring for people with mental health needs (Healthcare Commission 2007, Academy of Medical Royal Colleges 2008, Department of Health 2008, 2009). It also requires the general hospital to 'sign up' to the importance of training for all their staff. The authors found this co-operation was easier to achieve for the Liaison Practitioner employed within the acute Trust.

The authors adopted varying approaches, as follows, in the delivery of their educational strategies for the general hospital:

- Involvement in the induction programmes for new starters.
- Provision of formal study days: mental capacity, behavioural assessment and management, mental health disorders, risk assessment and management, etc.
- Provision of informal training with shadowing, staff listening to assessments or role modelling.
- One-hour sessions for medical staff as part of their training programmes: delirium, capacity assessment, behavioural management, etc.
- Unqualified staff skills sessions.
- Sessions of students on placements.
- Training with whole ward teams on safer handling of resistant patients.
- Training for senior managers on high level risk management.
- Accessing the general hospital staff into available training from the mental health trust.
- Training for volunteers on assisting with eating and drinking.

Whilst the research evidence base about the effectiveness of liaison interventions for older people is limited, evidence from mental health services working within bed-based intermediate care, or in residential and nursing care homes has relevance to Later Life Liaison Services; although there are obvious differences, there are more similarities than with Liaison Services of working age. Any alliance or collaboration that leads to a greater evidence base in support of Later Life Liaison Services is a positive step forward. The distinct model of care of these Liaison Services means that it is crucial that all Liaison Practitioners evaluate their role on an ongoing basis and collate their own data for service evaluations. Reviews arising from such evaluations help maintain the momentum to support developments and necessary expansion of services. Evaluation also provides feedback for the general hospital with regard to the work that has been completed in collaboration with staff and enables planning for action areas for the coming year.

Collecting data on the process factors that reflect the 'liaison' components of the roles is as important as routine outcome data. The authors ensured that evaluation was seen as a crucial element of their work, and was initiated as their services commenced.

Conclusion

This chapter described the application of an holistic person-centred model of care that the authors had been delivering within two very different general hospital settings. The high prevalence of older people with mental health needs in general hospitals, critical reports over the quality of care these patients receive, and the growing policy guidance in the field all require the urgent provision of effective multi-disciplinary Mental Health Later Life Liaison Services throughout the UK. Sadly, this objective still seems a long way off at the present time. What the authors hope to have demonstrated in writing this chapter is that sole Liaison Practitioners or small teams, whether employed within mental health or acute trusts, are able to make a difference to the quality of care that older people receive when admitted to a general hospital. This is only possible through the establishment and maintenance of collaborative working relationships with other Liaison Practitioners and with the general hospital staff across the whole organisation.

Acknowledgements

Lorraine Burgess

I would like to acknowledge Dr Ross Overshott, Liaison Consultant Psychiatrist, and Dr Paul Cohen, Older Age Psychiatrist, for their encouragement, guidance and support they offered me during my Dementia Nurse role in the Acute Hospital. Also the Older Age Physician Consultants at the University Hospital of South Manchester NHS Foundation Trust for having such faith in my work and role.

Helen Pratt

I would like to acknowledge the contribution and professional encouragement of Dr Robert Baldwin, Dr John Holmes, Elizabeth Matthews and Debbie Cavanagh, and also Dr Carol Ann McArdle, the medical and secretarial team (Pennine Care NHS Foundation Trust – Stockport), and Tracey Burgin and Carol Ainsworth (Pennine Care NHS Foundation Trust – Tameside).

References

Academy of Medical Royal Colleges (2008) *Managing urgent mental health needs in the acute trust: a guide for practitioners, for managers and commissioners in England and Wales*, London: Royal College of Psychiatrists.

Age Concern (2006) *Hungry to be heard. The scandal of malnourished older people in hospital*, London: Age Concern.

Alzheimer's Society (2007) *Dementia UK: A report into the prevalence and cost of Dementia, prepared by the Personal Social Services Research Unit (PSSRU) at the London School of Economics and the Institute of Psychiatry at King's College London for the Alzheimer's Society*, London: Alzheimer's Society.

Audit Commission and Healthcare Commission (2006) *Living well in later life. A review of progress against the National Service Framework for Older People*, London: Commission for Healthcare Audit and Inspection.

BAPEN (2003) '*Malnutrition Universal Screening Tool*' explanatory booklet. Available: www.bapen.org.uk (accessed 4 February 2010).

Berzins, K. (2004) 'Researching recovery from mental health problems', in S. Bradstreet and W. Brown (eds), *Scottish Recovery Network discussion paper 3*, Glasgow: Scottish Recovery Network.

Care Quality Commission (2008) *Criteria for assessing core standards in 2008/2009*, Acute trusts. Available: www.cqc.org.uk (accessed 4 February 2010).

Cheston, R. and Bender, M. (2000) *Understanding dementia. The man with the worried eyes*, London: Jessica Kingsley Publishers.

Department of Health (1999) *National Service Framework for Mental Health*, London: Department of Health.

——(2001) *National Service Framework for Older People: Modern Standards and Service Models*, London: Department of Health.

——(2003) *Community Care (Delayed Discharges) Act*, London: HMSO.

——(2005) *Securing better mental health for older adults*, London: Department of Health.

——(2008) *High quality care for all: NHS Next Stage Review final report*, London: Department of Health.

——(2009) *Living Well with Dementia: A national dementia strategy*, London: Department of Health.

Fielding, P. and Craig, L. (2007) *Independent review of older people's care at Tameside General Hospital*, Tameside: North West Strategic Health Authority.

Folstein, M.F., Folstein, S. and McHugh, P. (1975) 'Mini-mental state: a practical method for grading the cognitive state of patients for the clinician', *Journal of Psychiatric Research*, 12: 189–98.

Fossey, J. and James, I. (2008) *Evidence-based approaches for improving dementia care in care homes*, London: Alzheimer's Society.

Gill, P., Rigatelli, M. and Ferrari, S. (2007) 'Delirium', in G.G. Lloyd and E. Guthrie (eds), *Handbook of Liaison Psychiatry*, Cambridge: Cambridge University Press.

Health Advisory Service (1998) *Not Because They Are Old. An Independent Inquiry into The Care of Older People on Acute Wards in General Hospitals*, Brighton: Pavilion Publishing.

Health and Social Care Change Agent Team (2003) *Discharge from hospital: getting it right for people with dementia*, London: Department of Health.

Healthcare Commission (2007) *Caring for dignity. A national report on dignity in care for older people while in hospital*, London: Commission for Healthcare Audit and Inspection.

Holmes, J., Bentley, K. and Cameron, I. (2002) *Between two stools: psychiatric services for older people in general hospitals*, Leeds: University of Leeds.

Holmes, J. and House, A. (2000) 'Psychiatric illness predicts poor outcome after surgery for hip fracture: a prospective cohort study', *Psychological Medicine*, 30 (4): 921–29.

Hughes, J., Challis, D., Xie, C. and Bateson, J. (2007) *Delayed discharges from hospital. Discussion paper M197*, Manchester: PSSRU.

Inouye, S.K. (2000) 'Prevention of delirium in hospitalised older patients: risk factors and targeted intervention strategies', *Annals of Medicine*, 32: 257–63.

Inouye, S.K., Viscoli, C.M., Horwitz, R.I., Hurst, L.D. and Tinetti, M.E. (1993) 'A predictive model for delirium in hospitalised elderly medical patients based on admission characteristics', *Annals of Internal Medicine*, 119: 474–81.

Keady, J. and Hardman, P. (2010) 'Community Mental Health Nursing and Supportive Care', in J.C. Hughes, M. Lloyd-Williams and G.A. Sachs (eds), *Supportive Care of the Person with Dementia*, Oxford: Oxford University Press.

Kitwood, T. (1997) *Dementia reconsidered: the person comes first*, Buckinghamshire: Open University Press.

Lloyd, G.G. and Guthrie, E. (eds) (2007) *Handbook of Liaison Psychiatry*, Cambridge: Cambridge University Press.

Longson, D. (2007) 'Detection of psychiatric disorders in the general hospital: a practice guide', in G.G. Lloyd and E. Guthrie (eds), *Handbook of liaison psychiatry,* Cambridge: Cambridge University Press.

McCrone, P., Dhanasiri, S., Patel, A., Knapp, M. and Lawton-Smith, S. (2008) *Paying the price. The cost of mental health care in England to 2026*, London: King's Fund.

McNamara, P., Bryant, J., Forster, J., Sharrock, J. and Happell, B. (2008) 'Exploratory study of mental health: consultation-liaison nursing in Australia. Part 2. Preparation, support, role and satisfaction', *International Journal of Mental Health Nursing*, 17: 189–96.

Mayou, R. (2007) 'The development of general hospital psychiatry', in G.G. Lloyd and E. Guthrie (eds), *Handbook of Liaison Psychiatry*, Cambridge: Cambridge University Press.

Mental Health and Older People Forum (2008) *A collective responsibility to act now on ageing and mental health. A consensus statement issued by key organisations integral to the support, care and treatment of mental health in later life*, London: Mental Health and Older People Forum.

Minshull, P. (2007) *Age equality: what does it mean for older people's mental health services?*, North West Development Centre: Care Service Improvement Partnership.

National Audit Office (2007) *Improving services and support for people with dementia*, London: The Stationery Office.

National Institute for Health and Clinical Excellence (2004) *Self-harm: the short-term physical and psychological management and secondary prevention of self-harm in primary and secondary care*, London: National Institute for Health and Clinical Excellence.

——(2005) *The short term management of disturbed/violent behaviour in in-patient psychiatric settings and emergency departments*, London: National Institute for Health and Clinical Excellence.

——(2007a) *Anxiety: management of anxiety (panic disorder, with or without agoraphobia, and generalized anxiety disorder) in adults in primary, secondary and community care CG22*, London: National Institute for Health and Clinical Excellence.

——(2007b) *Depression: management of depression in primary and secondary care CG23*, London: National Institute for Health and Clinical Excellence.

National Institute for Health and Clinical Excellence/Social Care Institute for Excellence (2006) *Dementia: supporting people with dementia and their carers in health and social care. NICE clinical practice guideline 42*, London: National Institute for Health and Clinical Excellence.

Nuffield Council on Bioethics (2009) *Dementia: ethical issues*, London: Nuffield Council on Bioethics.

Packer, T. (1999) 'Attitudes towards dementia care: Education and morale in health care teams', in T. Adams and C.L. Clarke (eds), *Dementia care: Developing partnerships in practice*, London: Baillière Tindall.

Peplau, H.E. (1964) 'Psychiatric nursing skills and the general hospital patient', *Nursing Forum*, 3 (2): 28–37.

Pratt, H. and Ratcliffe, J. (2005) *Developing a Liaison Mental Health Service for older people within the general hospital: A good practice checklist for health and social care*, Care Services Improvement Partnership North West.

Ragaisis, K. (2005) 'Perspectives in psychiatric consultation liaison nursing. Bridging the gap', *Perspectives in Psychiatric Care*, 41 (4): 197–98.

Regel, S. and Roberts, D. (eds) (2002) *Liaison Mental Health – A Handbook for Nurses and Healthcare Professionals*, London: Baillière Tindall.

Roberts, D. (2002) 'Working models for practice', in S. Regel and D. Roberts (eds), *Liaison Mental Health – A Handbook for Nurses and Healthcare Professionals*, London: Baillière Tindall.

Roberts, D. and Whitehead, L. (2002) 'Liaison mental health nursing: an overview of its development and current practice', in S. Regel and D. Roberts (eds), *Liaison Mental Health – A Handbook for Nurses and Healthcare Professionals*, London: Baillière Tindall.

Royal College of Physicians and Royal College of Psychiatrists (2003) *The psychological care of medical patients. A practical guide. Report of a joint working party of the Royal College of Physicians and the Royal College of Psychiatrists*, (2nd edition), London: Royal College of Physicians.

Royal College of Psychiatrists (2005) *Who cares wins. Improving the outcome for older people admitted to the general hospital. Guidelines for the development of liaison mental health services for older people*, London: Royal College of Psychiatrists.

——(2008) *Rethinking risk to others in mental health services. Final report of a scoping group. College report 150*, London: Royal College of Psychiatrists.

Sharrock, J., Griggs, M., Happell, B., Keeble-Devlin, B. and Jennings, S. (2006) 'The mental health nurse: a valuable addition to the consultation-liaison team', *International Journal of Mental Health Nursing*, 15: 35–43.

Steis, M. and Fick, D. (2008) 'Are nurses recognising delirium? A systematic review', *Journal of Gerontological Nursing*, 34 (9): 40–48.

Stokes, G. (2000) *Challenging behaviour in dementia. A person-centred approach*, Oxon: Winslow Press.

Woods, R.T. (2001) 'Discovering the person with Alzheimer's disease: cognitive, emotional and behavioural aspects', *Aging & Mental Health*, 5 (suppl. 1): 7–16.

World Health Organization (1993) *ICD-10 Classification of Mental and Behavioural Disorders*, Geneva: World Health Organization.

11 Psychological interventions for complex and enduring mood disorders in older people

Struggling with a lifetime of depression

Stephen Davies

Key messages

- Chronic depression occurs regularly in late-life populations, often in phases with intervening periods of dysthymia (persistent low mood).
- How sadness is seen by the individual is as important as the biological and psychological symptoms of late-life chronic depression.
- Chronic depression often has its roots in traumatic earlier events and experiences.
- The chronically depressed older person has lived with a life-long depressed identity which masks the importance of these events to the person.
- Older people with chronic depression require a de-stigmatising, team approach to deal with their and their family's needs.
- A consistent caring 'secure base' from which to explore [their] problems is required.
- Psychosocial treatment of late-life depression is both possible and effective.

Introduction

Depression is usually characterised as the common cold of mental health problems. Statistics indicating the prevalence of depression and related key studies are described in Georgina Charlesworth and Janet Carter's contribution to this book (Chapter 4), so are not reiterated in detail here. Instead, I will focus on key models and psychological concepts that I have found helpful in understanding chronic problems of depression.

This chapter describes a composite case study, 'Mary', to illustrate the problems of chronic low mood in late life; she has to manage the vicissitudes of her current situation whilst also dealing with a legacy of psychological situations which have led to lifelong mood problems.

The problem of sadness and later life

Medically based models of mental health problems continue to dominate thinking about the people who have to live with the discomfort of these problems. This is particularly the case for people with complex or enduring forms of mental distress. Apart from the difficulties these people face with toxic labelling (Thornicroft 2006) inherent in stigmatisation (e.g. schizophrenia as shorthand for permanent dangerousness) and subsequent marginalisation, there is a general assumption that severity and chronicity of mental health problems must indicate neurobiological causation. This may be because it is more difficult to point to biological markers than in physical disease (e.g.

changes to tissue in heart disease) in order to make a diagnosis of an acute mental health condition in a convincing fashion. However, by defining mental health problems as entities which develop slowly and somewhat mysteriously (rather than by the action of numerous stressful events, for example), the illusion of an organic 'brain damage'-based account of chronic ill health can be maintained. An uneasy alliance is reached in stress-diathesis models of complex and enduring mental health conditions, but often in these models some form of biological supremacy is still implied with learning and social environment usually acting as trigger rather than pro-genitor of the condition. This puts attachment-related and recovery models of mental health problems at a disadvantage, although this disadvantage is to some extent self-imposed as these models may often use the dubious scientific backing of unproven psychoanalytic or sociological concepts.

People get depressed because bad things happen to them. They remain depressed because of the learning and memory implications of having bad things happen to them persistently throughout their lives. Cognitive psychology indicates that the brain is a messy, rather distracted worker rather than the chair of an organised and efficient committee, and it has far too much to do in any one day (Marcus 2008). Therefore, it embraces shortcuts to understanding with alacrity and gets it wrong quite often as a result. Some behavioural palaeontologists believe that *Homo sapiens* arose as the dominant hominid group because of excessive physiological reactions to stress, which now cause problems of over-reaction (Heckhausen 1999). This evolutionary imperative produces enough hits to ensure survival. However, in a world where direct physical threat of predation is reduced for most humans most of the time, it produces considerable problems with everyday life. The reliance on a Kraepelinian (after Emil Kraepelin) universe of symptom constellations pointing to underlying physical pathology is unnecessary. The most serious error that arises here is the misattribution of symptoms of psychological states which arise from loss events, to clearly delineated biological causation (Knight 2003). As these authors assert, in this model the client becomes an object for classification rather than an individual for investigation.

What does this literature say about the course of a complex and enduring mood problem which may have been with an older person for most of their life? First, it cannot be assumed that the classifications to which the client has been subjected are accurate. The system of labelling used has developed in a context-affected fashion and thus needs to be seen as being part of this history of psychiatry and not somehow separate from it. For example, the term 'schizophrenia' was used variably over the last century; some authors would say meaninglessly (Johnstone 1998). Thus you cannot necessarily compare the experience of two individuals with the same diagnosis, as such diagnoses are not very reliable (Bentall 2009). Second, the older people who now have complex and enduring mood problems may have been as much affected by this context as by any stable 'illness'. For example, the definition of depression and the moral tinge that adolescent behaviour could attract before the Second World War may have led to a number of outcomes such as hospitalisation, psychosurgery, electro-convulsive therapy (ECT) and various experimental medications and medical procedures. Chronic bouts of sadness relating to real and perceived losses may be mislabelled as major depressive episodes. In this way, episodes of sadness may become connected through the assumption of a common, underlying, biological fault, which may not actually be justified.

Basic biological theories are often promoted as being the best 'fit' for mental disorders. This is particularly the case for those mental health problems that are seen as complex or enduring in nature. As Szasz (2007) and Bentall (2004, 2009) indicate, the Kraepelinian theories of mental disorder which have so influenced psychiatric nosology over the last 100 years have governed thinking and research into discovering these processes. They provide useful 'evidence' for a classification that can be relied upon both by doctors and insurers to provide a coherent framework for research and payment, respectively.

Attachment theory

In many ways attachment theory, as proposed by John Bowlby (1969, 1973) initially in the early 1950s and formally in the late 1960s, was an idea that had a surprisingly difficult birth. The idea that children were not small adults, but different creatures in need of a special form of care was relatively new. Social change around children's care and treatment only really came into force with the introduction of compulsory education and the separation of work from childhood. Sigmund Freud's suggestion that children had a complex, instinct-based, internal life was treated as scandalous and misguided by many of his contemporaries (Masson 1988). However, particularly after the horrors of the First World War when civilised society descended into the most primitive savagery again, psychoanalysis became increasingly accepted in Western Europe. Possibly, after the trauma of war, there was a revived interest in the mental life of families and how individuals could be 'put back together' within them. Significant psychoanalysts such as Wilfrid Bion were Great War veterans and the association between exposure to traumatic events and emotional damage was clearly set in their minds.

Attachment theory did not start well. When Bowlby first presented his ideas there was considerable hostility from a psychoanalytic community that still wanted to believe in the primacy of very early, highly complex, intrapsychic phenomena based on conflict between drives, rather than more straightforward (and demonstrable) interpersonal processes between parent and child and later with society at large. Nonetheless, the results of Bowlby's work today are the closest thing that we have to a grand universal theory of psychopathology.

Why chronic mood disorder?

The brain in humans is designed to be as flexible as possible as a learning engine. The drawback of this evolutionary gamble is that the wrong things can be learned. Thus, vulnerable individuals are damaged mentally by their experiences. This damage is enshrined in the brain's neural and chemical reactions to extreme stress. Neurological and neurochemical learning and patterning as a result of early abusive and neglectful experiences may lead to later problems with emotional regulation, due to early learning of abnormal responses (Schore 1994, 2003, Simpson and Rholes 1998, Fonagy and Target 2002). These are lifelong effects, although there is some evidence that these abnormal responses can be attenuated and occasionally re-learned in reparative environments such as with loving, securely attached foster parents or an adult sexual partner (Clarke and Clarke 2003).

Bowlby predicted that attachment disruption in childhood would have two main effects on grown adults (Bowlby 1984). The most obvious consequence of such emotional disruption was the subsequent disruption of adult intimate relationships. Having to get close to others emotionally requires trust and regulation of emotional responses to intimate relationships. The key element of damaged attachment is deregulated emotional states. One of the most important forms of dysregulation is dissociation. The body has two well-known choices when responding to threat: to fight it or run away from it. However, this 'fight-flight' response is missing a third element which is often only deployed when the threat is inescapable or overwhelming. This 'freeze' response is used as a last resort to stay hidden or minimise the effects of injury. Children often select this response as they have little prospect of being able to fight or flee.

The team (this is a constructed description and situation)

As with most mental health services for older people the teams usually involved in such cases are: a community team made up of community psychiatric nurses (CPNs), occupational therapists, social workers and psychiatrists; and a ward team made up of the 'in-patient equivalent' of the aforementioned professions. The community team worked both with people with dementia and with people with mental health problems over the age of 65. The ward team worked on a unit for in-patient services for people with mental health problems over the age of 65. The ward was traditionally built, with bays for four and sixpatients, and some double and single rooms.

Both teams had produced some very well considered episodes of care for clients in often challenging financial and physical circumstances. The teams had less contact with each other than was thought optimal but this was often related to pressure of work rather than any particular animosity. The teams had somewhat different views of the causes of their clients' mental health problems, with the ward team tending to endorse the more biologically based, traditionally medical view.

The case

This is a constructed case and team, based on the author's clinical experience and designed to illustrate possible issues arising in this problem area.

Mary is a 78-year-old retired secretary who has been significantly sad in her mood since the death of her husband three years ago. When Mary's husband died from cancer she was initially unable to grieve for him and mainly felt numb. Her relationships with her children deteriorated as she isolated herself from them. The event which triggered her referral had actually begun as her having a row with her second daughter over the physical abuse of one of the latter's children. This daughter has a problem with alcohol and financial matters, and Mary had accused her of hitting one of her children. Social services had investigated a complaint by a neighbour relating to the neglect of the children by this daughter some years earlier and Mary had been unable to speak to her since. After this row, Mary had been found by a neighbour wandering in the town and had taken her to her general practitioner's (GP) surgery. Mary had been sent to A&E by her GP as she appeared to be in a confused and tearful state, stating that her daughter had been arrested for fraud. She calmed down quickly whilst at the hospital and told the duty psychiatrist that she had just been upset about her daughter's financial problems and had misconstrued these as fraud. The client remained very depressed and had talked of killing herself when seen for follow-up by her GP. As such, she was referred to the mental health team for older people.

The mental health team for older people discussed the referral and felt that the case was urgent as the client's daughter had rung the previous day to express her anxiety about her mother. When the client was phoned after the meeting she was reported as tearful and wanting to know 'when I will see the doctor again'. She was prioritised as an urgent case and two members of the team went to see her at her home.

Initial assessment

At this assessment the client appeared alternately calm and distressed with little sense of the reasons for this being ascertained by the team members. It emerged that her current problems had actually started about four-and-a-half years ago when the family next door had suddenly moved away. The client was very friendly with the mother of the family and with the three children, who called her 'granny'. It was rumoured that the family had had some problems with child protection and that the father had been accused of domestic violence to both wife and children. The client became very upset about this during the assessment, being very agitated that she should have seen something and done something about it.

Mary lives on her own in the house that she occupied with her family for nearly 30 years. She has four children: three daughters and a son. Her relationships with her two older children, her son, Mark, and daughter, Mandy, are distant and she has not seen them since the death of her husband. Claire, her third child, lives locally and it is Claire's children with whom Mary has the most contact. Her relationship with Claire is somewhat fraught on occasions and they argue over the care of Mary's grandchildren. Claire was divorced from a violent relationship some years before and Mary was always worried that the grandchildren might have been affected by the experiences inflicted on their mother. Claire has always refused to discuss the matter with her mother.

Mary feels that Claire is 'like me' and is worried that her legacy has somehow been transmitted to her child. She was also concerned that she was able to see her chronic problems with mood in her daughter and that she would somehow damage her grand-children. Mary felt responsible for this hypothesised damage and felt that she needed to 'watch my children all of my life' to see whether her problems with chronic depression would be visited on them. She said that on any occasion where her daughter or her grandchildren appeared to be upset she was convinced that this was because they had inherited her 'nervous problems', and it was only a matter of time before the weakness that she had as a result of her depression would become part of their lives.

The community team had undertaken a screening assessment at which the Mini-mental State Examination (MMSE; Folstein, Folstein and McHugh 1975) and the 15-item Geriatric Depression Scale (GDS-15; Yesavage *et al.* 1983) were administered. Mary scored well within the non-dementing range on the MMSE but her GDS score was well into the depressed range with a positive response to hopelessness and suicidal intent questions.

The community mental health team for older people were concerned about the level of 'harm to self' risk associated with Mary and there was a move on their behalf to have her admitted to hospital. They also reflected on the client's interactions with them, and asked for a consultation with the team psychologist to get them to think more about their relationship with this client. The psychologist and the team had previously discussed Mary in a weekly team meeting when considering the case management issues relating to her acceptance by the community team. Some months before, during a training session for the community team, the psychologist had presented the idea of the 'secure base' derived from the attachment theory of John Bowlby and operationalised in the 'BABI' (Brief Attachment Based Intervention) method described by Holmes (2003). In this intervention the team (and other institutions) are reacted to by the client in the same way as to attachment figures. They can provide and withdraw care and the client will react in an attachment-based way (dependent clinging or hostile rejection, for example) in response to these psychological actions of the team (Heard and Lake 2004). This reciprocation often forms the basis of the relationship between the client and the teams to which they relate.

Psychological assessment

The psychologist saw Mary for an assessment session at her GP's surgery as part of a primary care initiative and she completed a Beck Depression Inventory (Beck, Steer and Brown 1996), which yielded a score in the severely depressed range. The psychologist arranged to see Mary again at the mental health unit in order to begin a course of cognitive behaviour therapy (CBT) for depression. However, as the team began to work with the client (which involved some home visiting by staff and the prescription of various antidepressants, all of which were discontinued after a few days as Mary complained of side-effects), Mary rang the community team office in a distressed state to indicate that she felt very depressed and suicidal. One of the psychiatrists went to see her at home as a matter of urgency and she was admitted to the in-patient unit for older people with mental health problems.

Hospital admission

Within two days of admission, Mary was completely calm and wanted to return home. There was no sign of the extreme agitation and distress that she showed on admission. In the subsequent ward round the client's CPN explained to the team that Mary often feels overwhelmed by being on her own and this causes unbearable feelings of depression. At the same time, she said that she does not really understand how this happens and there are often rapid oscillations in the mood of the client. The ward team considered that the client might suffer from bipolar affective disorder and thought about medicating the client accordingly. Mary refused to take any medication and was keen to go home instead. She explained her rapid cycling in mood as a long-term phenomenon that she was 'just used to' and that these 'moods' had been with her for most of her life.

When Mary was on the ward there were times when she was almost catatonic, becoming very withdrawn in her room. ECT and medication were administered with little success and the ward team were relieved when Mary began to interact with other patients on the ward. She became particularly close to another frail patient on the ward with similar histories of chronic depression or dysthymia. This group increased in solidarity on the ward and formed an alliance when any one of them was due to be discharged. They resisted this as a group, pointing out flaws in discharge plans or community services. The ward staff reacted by branding the group as disruptive and dependent. Mary was identified as the 'ringleader' and there was increasing conflict between her and some ward staff as she refused to go on weekend leave or to participate in the ward's leave programme in general. The ward staff and doctors decided that Mary was ready for discharge and she was sent home.

Discharge treatment

The community mental health team was concerned about the discharge of the client from hospital and arranged a daily visiting programme to see her at home. They were very concerned about Mary's occasional episodes of distress and her feelings of wanting to kill herself. Their concern prompted two visits by psychiatric staff, who were unable to find any evidence of suicidal intent on their visits. Mary's mood and demeanour seemed to change somewhat depending on whom she was with. However, she said that she felt sad all of the time and that she felt 'nothing' quite a lot of the time.

The team were also puzzled as to why they felt so worried about her, as they knew that they had 'more serious cases' on their books. The pervasiveness of the client's depression and its chronicity seemed to be factors which affected them disproportionately. Maybe these were attachment-related phenomena having a secure base effect on the team and causing excessive worry in them? The team members felt that they needed to discuss this client more frequently with the psychologist than others.

When Mary came back into psychological therapy after her hospital stay there was much more discussion of how she felt. She said that she often felt like there was very little point in feeling better. She felt that she had always been sad and that one day differed very little from the next. She said that she found it difficult to get any satisfaction from any activities and that she had forgotten what feelings were now. She felt that this had been the situation for a very long time now and she expected little from her emotional life as a result. She felt that this had begun when the abuse at the hands of her father ceased around the age of 16, when she had left the household to live with an aunt.

Mary disclosed that she was beaten regularly by her father from the age of about six. She recalled that her father had wanted to assault her younger brother but she would 'draw his fire' by doing something that she knew would attract his ire. She remembered on one of these occasions her mother intervened when her father started to hit her with a stick that he had found in the garden. As Mary started to talk in therapy the process itself brought back the details of half-forgotten abuse episodes where she had suffered terrible physical harm at the hands of a violent, alcoholic father. She became infuriated with her mother who did nothing during these drunken rages, but then realised that her mother was often beaten herself and also tried to distract her husband's attentions from the younger children who could not take a beating. Mary's realisation of this allowed her to feel slightly less depressed, although she often ruminated about her mother. She felt that her mother was always depressed as a child and just 'kept herself to herself'.

As therapy progressed Mary was able to disclose more of her abuse legacy, her beliefs about herself and her depression. At the age of 11 her father began to become interested in her sexually and would usually assault her sexually when he was drunk. Mary had a very clear memory of hearing the front door close late at night when her father returned from drinking. She was able to tell from the force with which the door was closed whether she would 'have a visit' that night. These visits initially involved fondling through clothing and progressed to rape by the time Mary was 14. If she did not comply she was threatened with violence – to her or to her younger brother who had been badly beaten on several occasions for 'defiance'. When Mary was 12 she left school as her father, who was a tobacconist, insisted that he wanted her to work in the shop. Mary had been asked about why she was leaving school by one of the teachers with whom she had a good relationship, and she disclosed the physical abuse to which her mother, herself and her brother were subjected. The teacher was distressed by this disclosure and said that she would report it to the head teacher and that they would keep her in school. However, nothing happened and Mary was removed from the school the following month.

Mary recounted an incident that occurred when she was 14, which she felt was still very clear in her memory. She had suffered a brutal rape at the hands of her father the previous night and was required to work with him at the shop. He had gone to the pub for lunch and she was in the shop on her own when she became very distressed and decided to kill herself. The shop was on a busy main road and she walked out of it and ran without looking across this road. She felt at the time she definitely wanted to die but reached the opposite pavement without injury. At this point she felt a general feeling of numbness come over her where her feelings did not seem to be related to her situation. This she offered as her explanation for her chronic problems with depression. Most of the time Mary was unable to feel anything.

When Mary was 16 she left home after a particular sequence of events. Her father's drinking had lessened as he had fallen ill with a stomach complaint, the cause of which no one knew. Mary had struck up a friendship with the delivery boy from the grocer's shop a few doors away from her father's shop. Her father was in the shop less due to his illness and the friendship grew in intensity. She was asked out to the cinema by this young man and sought permission from her mother, knowing that her father would refuse. Her mother was happy with the arrangement but warned Mary not to tell her father.

The couple went to the cinema without event but she returned home to her furious father who had beaten Mary's whereabouts out of her mother after coming home early from the pub. He accused her of being a 'whore' and beat her with a fireside iron. He then tied her to a chair and cut off most of her hair. Mary became acutely distressed and her mother then took her to the doctor, who arranged for her admission to a local acute hospital for a few days for treatment of her physical injuries. Mary said nothing to the doctors when her mother insisted that she had fallen down the stairs. On discharge, she returned home, but was locked in her bedroom. About two days later the bedroom door was unlocked by her aunt, her mother's oldest sister, when her father was out, and she was given a hat to wear on the journey to her aunt's house at the other end of the country. Her aunt looked after her for several weeks while her hair grew back. During this time her father attempted to visit but was told that if he tried the police would be called. Mary remembered her mother coming to visit her on a few occasions but that she seemed distant and cold on these occasions.

At this point in therapy Mary recalled an event that she felt occurred when she was about four years old. Her mother took her and her younger brother, who was then about two, out shopping. She recalled her mother telling her and her brother to stay on one side of the road while she went into a shop on the other side and then described the phenomenon of holding her brother's hand in a 'sea of trouser legs'. This was a time when she felt close to her brother and it was one of the few times in therapy that she demonstrated any strong emotion. It was also one of the few things that she disclosed to other workers as she began to talk about her past.

Mary remained with her aunt until she was 18, when she was called up into the Auxiliary Territorial Service (ATS). She felt that the Second World War had had little impact on her up to this point because of her family circumstances. She had never seen the boy who took her to the cinema again, but knew that he was in the army. After training she was posted to a large army base where she worked in various administrative positions. She had a number of relationships at this time although she disliked sex and would only tolerate this if she felt that the relationship was casual and not likely to last. She said that this was easy to achieve as most of her relationships were with soldiers who were rapidly posted somewhere else. She also related an incident when she was found with a female colleague in bed in her hut. This led to threats of a court martial for both parties but Mary was required to attend the medical officer on the base instead for a while, which she said involved 'tea and a chat about the weather'. There was also some talk about admission to a psychiatric hospital as an alternative to court martial but this did not happen at that time as the case was dropped. Mary mentioned this event once briefly in therapy and refused to discuss it again.

Mary was demobbed from the ATS at the end of the war and went to work in a city office as a secretary. It was here that she met her husband and they married quickly at a local registry office without the knowledge of either family. They then moved to the city close to his relatives and lived a happy life there, having four children. Mary loved her husband very much, although she found sex to be uncomfortable and unsatisfying and was profoundly depressed after the birth of each child, leading to psychiatric hospital admissions after the births of her first two children and out-patient management after the third and fourth, all for depression. She gave her husband a limited account of her experiences and he assumed the depressions that she suffered regularly were something to do with her children rather than an abuse legacy.

The team's reaction

The team were initially shocked and angered by Mary's disclosures and expressed a great deal of sympathy for her symptoms and her situation. As Mary consented to allow them to know some information from her past they were able to form a more stable relationship with her. However, she still found it difficult to relate to her depression, which they also felt was a permanent medical condition. They also shared her worries about the depression being transmitted to her grandchildren in some genetic fashion. The team were able to understand the importance of providing a secure base for Mary and a protocol was established to allow this to happen with one person from within the team being available to visit and provide other communication consistently (this was before the largely administrative role of Care Co-ordinator was invented to replace clinical consistency) to and from the team. Mary really appreciated this although she continued to have persistent problems with dysthymia.

Mary continued to find living on her own difficult and regularly felt suicidal. The team struggled with the fact that there was little suitable provision for Mary in residential accommodation as the assumption is often that older people only require such accommodation when they have a significant level of dementia. Mary had found it very difficult to manage in the community since her husband's death and had liked being contained whilst on the hospital ward. As a result, both Mary and the team felt that she needed more containment and supervision and she went to live in a care home in a neighbouring town.

Mary found it difficult to settle in the care home, as the other residents were often confused and would come into her room at night which was a disastrous re-enactment of her abuse legacy. She felt more and more depressed in this home and wanted to kill herself regularly. Eventually she was re-admitted to hospital where it was felt that she needed ECT again. Once again the ward and community teams were in considerable conflict about this. One of the bridges that was built between these teams was through Mary attending a daily occupational therapy session where she did some artwork. Both the community and ward occupational therapy teams were able to help her with this, which she found cathartic and a way of explaining her past in a more psychological way. This therapy allowed the two teams to build a common narrative with Mary about her life, her experience of having a 'mental health problem' and of having a 'history of chronic depression'.

The psychologist was also able to re-engage Mary in a (CBT) oriented but narratively informed set of therapeutic conversations based on Moore and Garland's (2003) concept of working with chronic depression. This addresses the beliefs that develop in chronic depression around the permanent identification that the person has with being 'a depressive', the immutability of depression and the impossibility of recovery. Also important are the instillation of hope in the recovery process and the importance of life story and life review in developing a less restricted and self-critical view of the self and where it has been.

It may be that the story had to end and it was tragically or mercifully quick for Mary when it did. She had been feeling ill for a while before coming into hospital the second time. She had time to talk about it to the ward staff who asked her to see a specialist. A rare and rapidly advancing cancer killed her quite gently within four months. During this time she was able to say goodbye to her estranged daughter, saw her grandchildren, and died in a hospice with family there.

Different people knew different things in the team about Mary's last illness and her transfer to a hospice was a shock for some. The community team felt embarrassed and ashamed about not spotting her illness earlier. The ward team initially made them pay for it by denigrating the quality of psychological care provided by the community team, but then as Mary grew quieter so did they. The chronic sadness that Mary had lived with for so long finally came out in a series of informal discussions with staff.

It was felt at this time that both of the teams could usefully discuss the interaction between ward and community staff and a rotation of staff was discussed. Mary had also received a number of different diagnoses over her life with mental health services – bipolar affective disorder and schizoaffective disorder being two more recent ones. The teams were able to have a discussion about how to describe someone with chronic depression in the most helpful way. There was also a useful discussion between the clinicians about the use of medical treatments with individuals with chronic depression and how these could be combined with psychosocial approaches to understanding how to address such lifelong problems. In this way Mary's treatment brought elements of mental health care and the teams that operated them together in a new way for which they had not been originally designed. The categories that had been invented for professionals to understand and conceptualise the problems of people with mental health problems were largely unhelpful in assisting Mary. However, it was very helpful to all parties to reflect on the phenomenology of her distress and numbness, the feeling and experience of the chronic problems with depression that she had as a result of her traumatic and difficult losses.

Discussion

1 Attachment theory is relevant for people with depression across the life-span.

Bowlby (1969, 1973, 1984) developed the theory of attachment to account for the necessity of close relationships and the psychological damage caused by their disruption. As I have argued in relation to trauma, attachment relationships can be disrupted across the life-span (Davies 2001, 2006, 2008). It is remarkable that the significance of old age for attachment challenges is described only once explicitly. Hansson and Carpenter's (1993) concept of Relational Competence is the only coherent account of the attachment consequences of late life. Older people often face more separation and loss challenges in late life than the blinkers of institutional ageism allow society to contemplate. Relational Competence recognises past and present aspects. Past aspects are the interpersonal behavioural skills that the individual has acquired in childhood in the context of a secure and emotionally containing set of close relationships. Present aspects are the emotional regulation and behavioural skills needed for initiating and maintaining new relationships in the difficult context of loss and separation that old age brings. Attachment involves the emotional intelligence to regulate strong emotions and to react flexibly to loss and separation events. Later life can be very tough and is often made tougher by the gross ageism and emotionally ignorant context within which many older people live.

Bowlby (1984) predicted that the quality of and satisfaction with adult intimate relationships would be determined by attachment experiences, and that episodes of loss would be more problematic for those with less than optimal attachment experiences. There is some evidence that resilience can be built even in insecure attachment conditions and that Bowlby's predictions are probably over-specified. However, a bleak early environment can lead to chronic depression as the individual finds it difficult to use the models about others generated by their experiences to satisfy their need for attachment to others.

2   Teams are secure bases too.

Individuals are not the only aspects of the attachment equation in later life. Mental health teams can also act as secure bases for the often attachment-compromised people whom they serve. Holmes (2003) set out the mechanism by which this could happen for individuals but this could also be applied to teams. Holmes termed this process the BABI where the relationship with the client passes several different stages of development and there is re-enactment of the attachment relationship. Heard and Lake (2004) had previously considered the attachment implications of the caregiving relationship and produced some useful observations on how the caregiver–care receiver relationship works. For teams to act as parenting figures to either maintain or re-establish secure attachment interaction can be a delicate operation. However, to assume that any interaction between a team and an individual client does not have systemic consequences is also erroneous (Davies 2009). Consequences are the inevitable result of any human interaction, so the team's role with clients with chronic depression is likely to be critical or enabling. Teams can choose the latter in order to allow the positive attachment consequences of such contact and optimism to be introduced in the service of the recovery of the client. Also, in line with the emphasis on the self-in-healing that characterises the Recovery movement in mental health, this relationship can be used by the client as they wish.

3   Chronic depression is different in later life.

Most commentators have assumed that the psychological processes underlying depression are the same whether the person who suffers is doing so as part of an acute depression or is more related to a recurrent, chronic pattern of depression. However, some in the field are beginning to question this medicalised idea of depressive distress (McCullough 2000, 2006, Moore and Garland 2003). The key elements of these newer models of treating chronic depression are that the client develops a belief system about the depression, its operation, its history and its outcomes. Beliefs about the self as depressed, the inevitability of permanent dysthymia and episodes of major depression then become part of the individual's life. As such, these systems then perpetuate the dysthymia and the associated chronic depression risk. Mary found it difficult to address her chronic depression because she believed that no recovery was possible. She saw the nature of depression as fixed and immutable.

4 The role of institutional ageism in chronic depression in late life.

Ageism still dominates services and opportunities for older people. However, the more subtle, less conscious form of age discrimination, sometimes referred to as institutional ageism (Davies 2006) is even more prevalent as overt ageism is occasionally brought into question. This institutional form of age discrimination states that older people are inevitably going to be depressed by the very fact of being old. This concept of 'realistic depression' often becomes a guiding principle when interviewing or providing services for older people with mental health problems. This often paralyses the thinking of professionals involved with older people and treatment of depression is thus relegated to an inconsequential set of actions which are given little priority.

However, this professional paralysis is only part of the picture and possibly the lesser portion of the discrimination that keeps older people as an untreated, inferior group in modern Western societies. Self-stigmatisation by older people themselves of their ageing and their mental health may provide the single greatest barrier to the comprehensive and sustained treatment of older people with problems with chronic depression. Laidlaw *et al.* (2004) in their model of depression wisely included the context within which the depression of the older person is experienced. The person who has experienced chronic depression throughout their life with an often unshakeable feeling of dysthymia, is then confronted with the beliefs of their ageing generation as well as the beliefs of those who are younger. These beliefs may include the value of thought suppression and the disadvantage of discussing emotions. Such beliefs hardly make the environment conducive to an older person engaging in difficult and emotionally painful psychotherapy, or for a service providing a comprehensive, psychologically minded programme to assist in such a therapeutic endeavour. Institutional ageism seems to keep the public focused on dementia as the great problem of later life when it is often the misery of chronic mood disturbance, particularly depression, which may keep individuals from enjoying a decent quality of life and may even contribute to their premature death.

5 The use of systemic interventions in teamwork with chronically depressed older people.

Most of the treatment and intervention regimes used with Mary were based on an empirical approach to helping others. This approach is predicated on the assumption that observable phenomena, such as signs of disease, are the basis for treatment of depression. The person with chronic depression has arrived at late life with a legacy of poor biology and other internal imbalances which the ageing process has complicated as the body contributes further to the impossibility of definitive treatment. In this rush to restrain the biological inevitability of death, the psychosocial relationships between people attract less emphasis in team accounts of their clients than the internal physical relationships within their individual bodies. It is often the case that older people may live on their own or seem otherwise isolated, so that the assumption is made that they have no relationships. However, older people form a system that interacts with them in the same way as anyone else does (Davies 2009).

In what ways can the lives of older people with depression form a system with other interested parties? The team and Mary formed a system, often initially without really being aware of it. The parts of the system also formed around the two teams: the community team and the ward team and their relationships with each other and with Mary and her family. Part of this system was our attempt as a team to form a secure base to which Mary could relate. This basic form of interaction with others, based on availability of support and consistency in response, is key to a successful and informed psychological response by the mental health teams to the people with whom they work. The effective acknowledgement and use of these basic interaction requirements in the maintenance of human systems was an important part of the treatment process, even though it was often more intuitively led rather than explicitly used by the team. In a way, both teams were involved in a system of Mary's making, merely by her being involved with both services. This actually allowed both teams to begin to co-operate in a way that they had not thought about before coming into contact with Mary.

6   Mary's chronic depression, her life and her legacy.

Do people with chronic depression in late life ever get better? One of the most important findings in the literature in this regard is that depression in itself is no higher in incidence in later life than it is when clients are younger (Karle, Ogland-Hand and Gatz 2002, Kohn and Epstein-Labow 2006). It is the things that occur when one is older, such as bereavement, illness and changes in financial, social and housing status, that tend to contribute to higher rates of depression in older people (Licht-Strunk *et al.* 2009). It does seem more likely that individuals who have had a legacy of abuse as children, leaving lasting attachment damage and subsequent problems with chronic depression as adults, will have a larger mountain to climb in order to deal with the inevitable problems of late life. However, increased risk does not relate directly to vulnerability and it may be the specifics of those late-life challenges which reduce the ability to cope rather than the general issues of ageing (Knight 2003). One of the effective factors in Mary's treatment may just have been the co-ordinating listening response that the team was able to produce. This was both verbally, by being available to discuss attachment-related material, and non-verbally by modelling the necessary conditions of the secure base. Mary herself was able to participate and mould this process by interacting in different ways with the ward and community teams. She could be dependent by staying on the ward and testing the patience of the ward team and she could be independent by going home and worrying the community team.

Conclusion

What is obvious is that the problem with chronic and persistent depression in any life is just that: chronic and persistent. The particular problem with it in an older person's life is that it can be so at a point when time is running out. Persistent trauma and the legacy of chronic depression that such almost unspeakable events can bring can result in emotional numbness and dissociation. This often does not allow a full experiencing of the inevitable psychological phenomenon of later life – reviewing that life. A recovery-informed approach to Mary and her difficulties with chronic depression has to put the client's own experience of their 'disorder' at the centre of any clinical response. Psychological models of chronic and persistent depression such as those proposed by McCullough (2000) and by Moore and Garland (2003), provide a useful basis for action in therapy. In such cases the clinical team needs to develop strategies to deal with the individual's beliefs that have grown up around the nature and course of the depression, as well as the external events which may be afflicting them; but these in themselves are not enough to understand the nature of interaction between clients, their families and their carers. Attachment theory and systems theory may also contribute to understanding the client within their context. The basic damage inflicted on the self through an abusive past, as in Mary's case, creates the circumstances within which a fundamentally poor view of the self as worthy and effective may develop (Moore and Garland 2003).

What helped Mary in this case? Her depression scores came down as she disclosed her past and seemed to make some sort of sense of it. They then rose again as she faced her terminal illness. There were many things that she found difficult, such as any reminders of the abuse which she suffered. One night in the nursing home a confused man wandered into her room, got into bed with her and tried to have sex with her. Mary was able to guide this man out of her room again and never reported it to the nursing home staff. She only told the community team several weeks later. It seemed that this event may have actually precipitated her re-admission to hospital as she said that she slept very little at night after this event. One simple solution could have presented itself: Mary could have been given the key to her room. However, this was not company policy and no one was certain where the room keys were kept. As psychologists and team working with people with complex mood and other problems we may think that our clients require complex interventions. However, sometimes the key is just the key.

References

Beck, A.T., Steer, R.A. and Brown, G.K (1996) *Manual for Beck Depression Inventory II (BDI-II)*, San Antonio, TX: Psychology Corporation.
Bentall, R. (2004) *Madness Explained*, London: Penguin.
——(2009) *Doctoring the Mind: Why Psychiatric Treatments Fail*, London: Penguin.
Bowlby, J. (1969) *Attachment*, London: Penguin.
——(1973) *Separation*, London: Penguin.
——(1984) *The making and breaking of affectional bonds*, London: Penguin.
Clarke, A. and Clarke, M. (2003) *Human Resilience: A Fifty year quote*, London: Jessica Kingsley publications.
Davies, S. (2001) 'The long-term psychological effects of traumatic wartime experiences on older adults', *Aging & Mental Health*, 5 (2): 99–103.
——(2006) 'Not Now Dear: Some Psychological effects of Institutional Ageism', *The Old Age Psychiatrist*, 41 (1): 7.
——(2008) 'Psychological Trauma: Assessment, Conceptualisation and Treatment', in R. Woods and L. Clare (eds), *Handbook of Clinical Psychology of Ageing*, 2nd edition, Chichester: Wiley.

——(2009) 'Systemic Therapy with Older People', in H. Beinhart, P. Kennedy and S. Llewelyn (eds), *Clinical Psychology in Practice*, Oxford: Blackwell Publishing.

Folstein, M.F., Folstein, S. and McHugh, P. (1975) 'Mini-mental state: a practical method for grading the cognitive state of patients for the clinician, *Journal of Psychiatric Research*, 12: 189–98.

Fonagy, P. and Target, M. (2002) *Mentalisation*, London: Allen Unwin.

Hansson, M. and Carpenter, A. (1993) *Relationships in Old Age*, New York: Guilford.

Heard, A. and Lake, P. (2004) *Attachment and Caregiving*, London: Routledge.

Heckhausen, J. (1999) *Developmental Regulation in Adulthood*, Cambridge: Cambridge University Press.

Holmes, J. (2003) *Attachment theory and Psychotherapy*, London: Routledge.

Johnstone, L. (1998) *Psychiatry and Anti-Psychiatry*, London: Penguin.

Karle, M., Ogland-Hand, S. and Gatz, M. (2002) *Assessing and Treating Late-Life Depression: A Casebook and Resource Guide*, New York: Basic Books.

Knight, R. (2003) *Psychotherapy with Older Adults*, New Jersey: Sage publications.

Kohn, R. and Epstein-Labow, G. (2006) 'Courses and outcomes of depression in the elderly', *Current Psychiatry Reports*, 8, (1): 34–40.

Laidlaw, K., Thompson, L.W. and Gallagher-Thompson, D. (2004) 'Comprehensive conceptualization for cognitive–behavioural therapy for late life depression', *Behavioural and Cognitive Psychotherapy*, 32: 389–99

Licht-Strunk, E., van Marwijk, H., Hoekstra, T., Twisk, J., de Hann, M. and Beekman, A. (2009) 'Outcome of depression in later life in primary care: Longitudinal cohort study with year's follow-up', *British Medical Journal*, 338: a3079.

McCullough, J. (2000) *Treatment for Chronic Depression: Cognitive Behavioral Analysis System of Psychotherapy*, New York: Guilford Press.

——(2006) *Treating Chronic Depression with Disciplined Personal Involvement*, New York: Springer.

Marcus, J. (2008) *Kluge*, London: Faber and Faber.

Masson, J. (1988) *The Assault on Truth*, New York: Penguin.

Moore, R. and Garland, A. (2003) *Cognitive therapy for chronic and persistent depression*, New York: John Wiley and Sons.

Schore, A.N. (1994) *Affect regulation and the origin of the self: the neurobiology of emotional development*, Hillsdale, NJ: Erblaum.

——(2003) *Affect regulation and the repair of the self*, New York: W.W. Norton.

Simpson, J.A. and Rholes, W.S. (1998) *Attachment and Close Relationships*, New York: Guilford Press.

Szasz, T. (2007) *Coercion as Cure*, Washington, DC: APA books.

Thornicroft, G. (2006) *Stigma*, Oxford: Oxford University Press.

Yesavage, J.A., Brink, T.L., Lum, O., Huang, V., Adey, M.B> and Leirer, V.O. (1983) 'Development and validation of a geriatric depression screening scale: A preliminary report', *Journal of Psychiatric Research*, 17: 37–49.

Part 3
A way forward

12 Key messages in later life mental health care

New directions and new ambitions

John Keady and Sue Watts

Introduction

In the Introduction to this book, we stated that our aim was to link the work of multi-disciplinary services with realistic evaluations of the complexities of living with mental health needs in later life. In the final production of the book, this link was pre-dominantly illustrated through detailed case study work where the specialism of the multi-disciplinary team, such as psychosis in later life (Chapter 5), was the diagnostic focus and the person living with the condition the focus of care. In order to tie the book together, this brief concluding chapter distils the key messages of the text to help shape thinking and debate in later life mental health practice.

Through the editorial process, four key messages emerged that transcended each chapter to provide a cohesive link throughout the book; we have named these four key messages as: 1 Biographical Mapping; 2 Integrative Team Working; 3 Generating an Evidence Base; and 4 Challenging Stigma. In addition, each of the four key messages has been ascribed five challenges that summarise our aspirations for new directions and new ambitions in later life mental health care. Naturally, these four key messages and five challenges are not the final word on the topic; rather, we see them as stepping stones for consensus to emerge, which, in turn, can help bridge reflection and practice change.

Key message 1: biographical mapping

Given the instructions to authors for the development of their chapters, it is perhaps no surprise that the older person's voice and lived experience is heard throughout the book. That was our intention, as mental health work across the life-span is all about people and their lives, relationships, social circumstances, beliefs, values and culture. To lift a person out of the context of their life story is to fragment a life. This was acknowledged in the *New Horizons* report (Department of Health 2009a), and it has been known for some time that a biographical approach to mental health practice is essential if shared decision-making and meanings are to guide intervention (Butler 1963, 1975, Johnson 1986). Indeed, as Bury (1982) himself identified nearly 30 years ago, chronic and adverse events experienced during the life course will cause a biographical disruption for the individual and this disruption is assimilated into the person's identity. Arguably, the work of mental health services and practitioners is to then identify, recover (where possible) and heal such a fracture. Grounding understanding and intervention within a biographical approach was seen repeatedly in this book. To take but one example, the work of Karin Terri Smith and Lorna Mackenzie of the Newcastle Challenging Behaviour

Team, outlined in Chapter 9, demonstrated the importance of knowing who Rebecca is/was in order to make sense of her presented behaviour and communication pattern. Without knowing Rebecca, the intervention and case formulation that was then enacted would be meaningless and rooted only in a professional construction of need.

Older people living with mental health needs have a significant part to play in developing and shaping their own care agenda. Indeed, each chapter in the book revealed rich and varied personal biographies that informed care practice with teams (and individuals within teams) working hard to locate the meaning of their intervention so that it was co-terminus with the understanding of the person living with the condition. As Richard Ward and his colleagues described in the opening chapter, from the perspective of older mental health service users effective participation in mental health practice is likely to be co-created. Consequently, the determinants of a successful intervention will be layered with the multiple meanings that this has for the person living with the condition. Spending time to map a person's biography, in whatever way possible, becomes a cornerstone of mental health practice in later life; without it, clinical decision-making is not personalised and, instead, is reduced to narrow generic diagnosis-based packages operationalised through custom and practice. What becomes unclear is how this biographical mapping then travels with the older person in the journey through their condition(s) and/or is used to inform future care planning. Perhaps this is a next step in clinical decision-making.

New directions and new ambitions – five challenges:

- To undertake biographical mapping with the person's involvement (wherever possible).
- To ensure that biographical mapping is central to case formulation, intervention and practice.
- To share and negotiate ownership of the biographical map.
- To define the constituents of a successful intervention through the person's own language and constructions, wherever possible.
- To explore and test the longitudinal use of biographical mapping in a recovery approach to later-life mental health practice.

Key message 2: integrative team working

The book has contained some inspiring examples of team working and functioning; for instance, the Croydon Memory Service (Chapter 8) and their illustration of a flattened hierarchical structure in order to produce a more blended, homogenous and accessible service. In short, it is the professional skills that are the important issue, not the professional undertaking the work. In the United Kingdom (UK) this new way of working is reflected in mental health policy (Department of Health 2005, 2007, 2009a) and in an overall consensus that blended team working works and is seen as a good thing. As Susan Benbow and her team shared during their chapter (Chapter 5), an advantage of a dedicated older people's community mental health team is the accumulation of a shared knowledge of common presentations in later life. Thus, the build-up of case knowledge (Liaschenko and Fischer 1999) becomes an important and necessary function of team practice and, de facto, of the individual operating within that team.

If one of the defining characteristics of successful team working is efficient record keeping, then it appears, in the UK at least, that there is still a long way to go.

Drawing once more on Susan Benbow and her team's contribution (Chapter 5), it was dispiriting to read that nursing and occupational therapists have the same records within the team, but that social care use different ones. Similarly, for this team, health and social care computers failed to talk to one another, thus adding an extra layer of complexity upon a service attempting to deliver and co-ordinate mental health care to a vulnerable population. Is it too naive to ask why, especially when organisational transparency and shared decision-making are cornerstones to upholding service quality? A part solution to this dilemma was found in Chapter 6 of the book when Rahul (Tony) Rao, Rachael Buxey and Kadiatu (Kadia) Jalloh called for an electronic record of intervention to be held. This would seem a sensible suggestion. Moreover, given the rise of the voluntary and third sector involvement in future service provision and support for older people with mental health needs, the necessity to find a workable solution to such territorial disputes becomes ever more pressing.

Effective team working rests on a shared vision, leadership, effective communication and practice learning (Doel and Shardlow 2009), yet few examples were shared in this book of teams training together. Perhaps this is simply our fault as Editors in not stressing the importance of sharing this process in our background notes to authors. All too often preparation for professional practice is about individual disciplines coming together for the first time with the expectation that case knowledge will somehow be enough to see things through. Once more, it would seem more thought and planning is required.

New directions and new ambitions – five challenges:

- To share case formulation, documentation and support/operational systems within everyday practice.
- To regularly find time for later life mental health teams to build a cohesive identity and effective working relationship.
- To develop a role for health education and health promotion within daily practice.
- To develop a strategy for shared practice learning and team supervision.
- To implement a research and evaluation component of practice work into team functioning.

Key message 3: generating an evidence base

A message that was heard consistently in the book was that practice-based research evidence was sparse and in need of development. Even in dementia care, where a *National Dementia Strategy* (Department of Health 2009b) exists, it would be natural to assume that a broad range of multidisciplinary services offering both pharmacological and psychosocial interventions for all stages of dementia is available in all areas of England; sadly, this is not the case (National Audit Office 2007). Indeed, the literature suggests that evidence-based psychological interventions in dementia are difficult to achieve in practice and are only in a formative state (Woods *et al.* 2003, Moniz-Cook *et al.* 2008, Keady and Hardman 2010). That is not to say that the care for older people with mental health needs is of poor quality; the case studies in this book, as well as our practice experience, would challenge this assumption. No, rather it is to say that the weight of 'gold standard' research evidence in mental health care, as generated through randomised controlled trials, has not been fully directed towards later life mental health care and services, a point that was also made by the Mental Health and Older People Forum (2008). A further complication in later life care is that the randomised controlled trial usually targets a unitary condition and excludes people with co-morbid conditions. Thus, information is extracted from clinical trials that may only be applicable to a small number of patients seen by clinical teams operating in the 'real world' of clinical service delivery. More diverse research methodologies are necessary to develop the knowledge base, including the contribution of older mental health service users to the process (Nolan *et al.* 2007).

Many older people's services have also been designed on the basis of a division between 'physical' and 'mental' health and 'organic' versus 'functional' mental health problems. Often these distinctions are artificial and do not reflect the complex reality of older people's health and well-being. For example, within this book, the mental health and later life liaison service chapter by Helen Pratt and Lorraine Burgess (Chapter 10) exposes the limited skills sets of adult nursing staff working in hospital acute care. As in the name of an earlier report, mental health remains '*Everybody's Business*' (Department of Health and Care Service Improvement Partnership 2005) and it is essential that this is reflected in core professional training.

New directions and new ambitions – five challenges:

- To influence research councils to fund randomised controlled trials across the spectrum of mental health and later life conditions.
- To place a responsibility on multidisciplinary teams and practitioners to conduct research in practice, and publish the results.
- To provide older people with mental health needs and family carers an opportunity to meaningfully contribute towards evidence generation.
- To ensure that research is conducted on social care interventions.
- To direct research towards professional training and extending professional skills sets.

Key message 4: challenging stigma

Calls to remove discrimination from service provision for older people have sometimes been accompanied by proposals that specialist mental health services for older people should be abolished in favour of generic provision for all ages, or that specialist dementia care can be separated from functional care for older people, for instance (see also Mental Health and Older People Forum 2008). Arguably, this is indirect discrimination arising from a narrow interpretation of anti-discrimination principles. Mental health problems in later life may be inextricably related to the onset or continuity of chronic illness, or to the life changes that are common in old age such as the psychological distress associated with ill-health and bereavement. Individuals with life-long severe and enduring mental health problems, as outlined so eloquently by Stephen Davies in Chapter 11 of this book, are by no means immune to any or all of the foregoing conditions. As Chapters 7 and 9 in this book also demonstrated, older people with cognitive impairment or dementia may also be depressed or anxious. Indeed, it is increasingly suggested that the stigma associated with dementia has been a major impediment to the development and uptake of effective services. In our youth-obsessed society, age and dementia are compounded to produce a formidable double stigma (Benbow and Reynolds 2000).

In many ways, this debate returns full-circle to the book's Introduction, where it was highlighted that stigma is the priority issue in mental health and later life care across the European Union (Jané-Llopis and Gabilondon 2008). Navigating a meaningful path to this goal is a complex task and one which will require a significant societal, cultural and historic shift in attitudes if it is to be achieved. A starting point would be a more robust and systematic public health and education campaign about mental health and later life. At present, such initiatives in the UK are woefully inadequate, fuelled by a public narrative (Somers 1994), which aligns 'mental health' to 'madness', and 'older people' to 'a drain on resources'. Arguably, to have depression and be lonely in old age is a cultural expectation not an exceptional state of affairs. Permanently replacing such public narratives with more active and inclusive representations of old age is a challenge, but one that is ultimately necessary if the stigma attached to older people with mental health needs is to be diminished and its influence weakened.

New directions and new ambitions – five challenges:

- To co-ordinate effective public health and education campaigns.
- To focus on mental well-being, improvement, personalisation and self-care.
- To instil positive images of ageing in the public mindset.
- To be aware of language and its continuation of stereotypes.
- To be aware of how we contribute to the perpetuation of stigma.

Conclusion

In the Introduction to the book we posed a question for mental health care and later life practice: where do we want to go? Chapters in this text have revealed a direction of travel and a reality that is practised day-by-day throughout the UK and, we would assume, elsewhere in the world. Some issues stand out and were summarised in our four key messages. Others are more hidden, with the voice of the older person still too silent in the mental health discourse to be fully and effectively heard. Undoubtedly, services need to develop better public health and education about mental health and later life. In all likelihood, a focus on personalisation, prevention, self-care and well-being will be the pattern of a new service configuration and commissioning structures for later life mental health services. Outcome measures will continue to rise in importance and technology will make an increasing contribution to self-care and care planning. Adaptation will be a key to unlocking the changing organisational structures and ever-diminishing resource allocation. Throughout this uncertainty one thing remains certain: namely, that mental health does not stand apart from a person's identity and sense of self but, rather, is integrated into the whole human being. The suffix to our book's title is 'Delivering an Holistic Model for Practice'; this remains our own clarion call for later life mental health services informed by the authors who shared their experiences in this text.

Thank you for reading this book.

References

Benbow, S.M. and Reynolds, D. (2000) 'Challenging the stigma of Alzheimer's disease', *Hospital Medicine*, 61: 174–77.

Bury, M. (1982) 'Chronic illness as biographical disruption', *Sociology of Health and Illness*, 4: 167–82.

Butler, R.N. (1963) 'The life review: an interpretation of reminiscence in old age', *Psychiatry*, 26: 1.

——(1975) *Why survive? Being old in America*, New York: Harper and Row.

Department of Health (2005) *New ways of working for psychiatrists: Enhancing effective, person-centred services through new ways of working in multidisciplinary and multiagency contexts*, London: Department of Health.

——(2007) *Mental health: New ways of working for everyone: Developing and sustaining a capable and flexible workforce*, London: Department of Health.

——(2009a) *New Horizons: A shared vision for mental health*, London: Department of Health.

——(2009b) *Living Well with Dementia, a National Dementia Strategy*, London: Department of Health.

Department of Health and Care Service Improvement Partnership (2005) *Everybody's Business: Integrated Mental Health Services for Older Adults: a service development guide*, London: Department of Health.

Doel, M. and Shardlow, S. (eds) (2009) *Educating Professionals: Practice Learning in Health and Social Care*, Hants: Ashgate Publishing.

Jané-Llopis, E. and Gabilondon, A. (eds) (2008) *Mental Health in Older People. Consensus paper*, Luxembourg: European Communities. Available: www.ec-mental-health-process.net (accessed 4 February 2010).

Johnson, M.L. (1986) 'The meaning of old age', in S.J. Redfern (ed.), *Nursing Elderly People*, London: Churchill Livingstone.

Keady, J. and Hardman, P. (2010) 'Community Mental Health Nursing and Supportive Care', in J.C. Hughes, M. Lloyd-Williams and G.A. Sachs (eds), *Supportive Care of the Person with Dementia*, Oxford: Oxford University Press.

Liaschenko J. and Fischer A. (1999) 'Theorizing the knowledge that nurses use in the conduct of their work', *Scholarly Inquiry for Nursing Practice*, 13: 29–41.

Mental Health and Older People Forum (2008) *A collective responsibility to act now on ageing and mental health. A consensus statement issued by key organisations integral to the support, care and treatment of mental health in later life*, London: Mental Health and Older People Forum. Available: www.mentalhealthequalities.org.uk/silo/files/consensus-statement-august.pdf (accessed 4 February 2010).

Moniz-Cook, E., Elston, C., Gardiner, E., Agar, S., Silver, M., Win, T. and Wang, M. (2008) 'Can training community mental health nurses to support family carers reduce behavioural problems in dementia? An exploratory pragmatic randomised controlled trial', *International Journal of Geriatric Psychiatry*, 23: 185–91.

National Audit Office (2007) *Improving services and support for people with dementia*, London: The Stationery Office.

Nolan, M., Hanson, E., Grant, G. and Keady, J. (eds) (2007) *User Participation in Health and Social Care Research: voices, values and evaluation*, Maidenhead: Open University Press/McGraw Hill.

Somers, M.R. (1994) 'The narrative constitution of identity: a relational and network approach', *Theory and Society*, 23: 605–49.

Woods, R.T., Wills, W., Higginson, I.J., Hobbins, J. and Whitby, M. (2003) 'Support in the community for people with dementia and their carers: a comparative outcome study of specialist mental health service interventions', *International Journal of Geriatric Psychiatry*, 18: 298–307.

Index

Bold page numbers indicate figures and tables. The index does not include all cited works and authors. Readers needing a complete list of works cited should consult the reference lists at the end of each chapter.

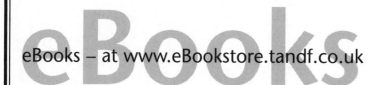